WEIGHT IS NOT THE PROBLEM:

A Non-Diet Approach to the Alchemy of Physical Transformation

Melanie Ezell

For Grandma Dona, who taught me that even grandmas can be swimsuit models.

My deepest thanks to Beth Lee for your dedication to this project and your friendship to me during some of my life's most pivotal moments. Thank you to my Mom for flying across the world multiple times to play with tractors on the floor and fly model airplanes with a two-year-old.

Table of Contents

Introduction

Body Alchemy is like a diet in only *one* way. It is a formula. When you take it step by step and do the work, you will see the results. But unlike a diet, there won't be any rules to follow. It won't take any willpower. You won't give up anything you love. You won't do workouts you don't enjoy. You won't even have to go around hungry. In fact, doing any of those things is only going to slow down your results. Body Alchemy is for anyone interested in losing weight without the pain of giving up the foods they love or being on a diet. Emotional eaters, binge eaters, and those that cannot seem to find the bottom of their endless hunger will find the tools and strategies here to solve the root of all overeating so they can finally give up the struggle and find a healthy body that they love

When I lost ten pounds in two weeks without trying, and another twenty-five pounds over the course of three months, all without changing my diet or lifestyle, I knew I had finally cracked the code. Before this, I struggled with weight (to the point of a clinical eating disorder and exercise addiction) for over fifteen years. I remember being so tired from a calorie-restricted diet that I wrecked a car, weighing and measuring every morsel of food that went into my body for years, month long juice fasts, and endless hours of brutal exercise. And still, every time I managed to lose some weight, it came back.

Now my weight is completely stable. If I lose a few too many pounds, my appetite gets strong, and I gain those pounds back. If I gain a few too many pounds, then my appetite drops, and I lose the weight. There is zero willpower involved. I never fight cravings. No more eating in secret, no more hiding wrappers in the trash before my husband sees them, no more packing my diet compliant meal for parties, no more fear of buffet tables. And the best part, not only is my weight in the healthy range, but I absolutely love my body. I like to try on clothes, I like to get dressed up, and I like to wear a bathing suit. I feel confident in my own skin. The freedom of looking at a menu and ordering what sounds good, of enjoying a guilt-free ice cream with my son, of walking by a store window and liking what I see, of waking up in the morning and not thinking about food—that kind of freedom—is like crossing over from hell into heaven. When this system clicked for me, I knew I had to share it with everyone.

So what is the secret I discovered that took me from being stuck in diet and exercise prison to being healthy and in love with my body without giving up my favorite foods or enduring painful workouts? What I'm about to say is going to sound crazy, so stick with me. There is nothing wrong with your weight. Nor is there anything wrong with the way you eat. Weight and food are symptoms. Think of them like the check engine light in your car. It is there for your benefit. When this light comes on, we would be fools to rush to a mechanic and beg them to turn off the light. Instead, we ask the mechanic to diagnose and fix the problem. Once the repair is done, the light automatically switches off. Similarly, once we've addressed the reasons our body is asking for food above and beyond what we need to maintain a healthy weight, then excess hunger will fall away, and our bodies will naturally take their healthiest shape and size. So this is the secret: body transformation is the effortless side effect of treating the root cause of excess weight. The root cause is much deeper than just a physical problem. It is mental, emotional and spiritual as well.

Diets treat only the symptoms; they shut off the check engine light without actually fixing the problem. This is precisely why diets don't work. Studies show 95% of dieters will regain their weight (Mann 2007). Restricting calories or denying oneself the simple pleasure of certain foods, such as carbohydrates, doesn't work to promote long term weight loss. It often works at first, but eventually the weight comes back. Given enough time, people under torture will cave. When we torture ourselves through diets and brutal workout routines, eventually the willpower runs out. Willpower is a finite resource; it always runs out. A starving animal will do anything, ANYTHING, to eat. When we restrict ourselves for long enough, our bodies will take over and we will eat, and generally the higher calorie the food, the better! That is when we find ourselves elbow deep in a tub of ice cream. Or if you are like I was, kneeling on a pee-covered gas station bathroom floor to purge what I had just binged on. That was torture. Not only do diets fail to achieve their goal of permanent weight reduction, but they are fundamentally unkind because they ask us to deny our basic needs.

Today many frustrated dieters are familiar with Intuitive Eating, a method highly touted in social media by anti-diet dieticians. Intuitive Eating teaches to allow all foods in all quantities based on listening to the body's natural intuition about what and how much to eat. On the surface, this seems like a much kinder way to treat one's body. And to those of us who understand that bodies are not flawed and instead are fully capable of supporting life, this sounds pretty good!

But there are a few problems here. The first is that food is engineered to be addictive. Before the invention of factory farming, worldwide shipping, and a whole host of processed foods, the only access to say, cherry pie, was when Grandma made one at Christmas. The cherries in the pie she had picked and then canned last summer; the flour for the crust came from wheat her neighbor grew in his field and ground into flour; the butter she churned from milk from the family cow she milked last night; and there was no sugar added because sugar was expensive, and cherries are already sweet!

But after World War II, our food supply system and food itself made a huge turn for the worse with the industrialization of food. Now, in most parts of the world, highly palpable and addictive food is available twenty-four/seven within walking distance. (But most Americans will drive because walking too has become a terrible inconvenience to speed and progress.) Many major food corporations have scientists on staff to engineer their food to be highly addictive. It is given the perfect amount of sugar, salt, crunchiness, or softness so that the brain becomes hijacked. One study found that the sugar changes dopamine levels and binds to opioid receptors. It even changes mRNA expression (Avna 2009). And it's not just big companies making processed foods that are exploiting these facts. My own mother loves to cook and host dinner parties. Everyone knows her food is fabulous and none of us miss a chance to show up at her house for her home cooking. We are addicted to her cooking. And it is no wonder. She taught me to cook by adding heavy cream to the soups, massive amounts of salt to the meat, butter and cheese on all the veggies, and sugar in almost everything. Any menu at any chain restaurant will have been designed with these same principles to keep you coming back. We are dealing with a real addiction problem, and it is no wonder weight-related illnesses plague the entire world and well-meaning women fail every diet out there only to end up "letting themselves go." Because food has become so much more than fuel.

Food is comfort. Food is pleasure. Food is distraction. Food is something to do. Food is stress relief. Food is a relief from social anxiety. Food is a sleeping pill. Food is a remedy for sleep deprivation and exhaustion from overworking, over producing, and overdoing. Food is a drug and all of us have used it that way from time to time.

And this is why going on a diet won't work. It is like telling an addict to simply stop using methamphetamine or an alcoholic to simply stop drinking. I have never met an alcoholic or drug addict who used the substance because of the way it tastes. No, the addict uses drugs and the alcoholic drinks to excess because they want to change the way they feel. They are struggling and the drug or the drink brings them temporary relief. "There is a significant overlap between mental health [conditions] and substance misuse, with over 80% of individuals having both," says Dr. Monty Ghosh, Addiction Specialist.

And the way we use food is no different. People suffering from depression, anxiety, PTSD, and more will temporarily receive a great deal of relief in a binge. I have always called food the drug for "good girls" since it is legal, necessary, and free from stigma. But you don't have to have a diagnosable condition to get temporary comfort from food. When we are sad, lonely, angry, hurting, worried, stressed, or confused, we use food to relieve the suffering from these powerful emotions. This is called emotional eating. And we have all done it!

So binge eating and emotional eating help us with our mental and emotional health, temporarily. But in the end, they cause bigger problems. And that is why diets will never cure the problem. They are like shutting off the warning light on a car's dashboard. It fixes the annoying dinging but never addresses the real problem . Eventually, it cannot be ignored.

Likewise, Intuitive eating is going to become an excuse to continue binging and emotional eating. Your intuition, in the form of sore joints and low energy and a body you loathe, is already telling you to slow down at the dinner table. But still, somehow you find it impossible to stop. You can try your darndest to listen to your intuition, but when food is your main way of coping with the harsh reality of being alive, you won't hear much above the cravings for highly palatable food. The intuition around what, when and how much to eat is no longer intuition about how to nourish a body, but rather intuition about how to cover over the pain of being human. Undoubtedly, your deeper intuition tells you that eating as much as you want of anything you want is going to lead to some increasing health issues and weight gain.

That is because food is not the problem. Here is the key. The *cravings* to eat more than what we need are the true problem. End the cravings, end the overeating.

After fifteen years caught in the diet cycle, including the last five years with clinical bulimia, I swore off diets all together and immersed myself fully in intuitive eating. I followed all the rules perfectly. And I gained fifty pounds, thirty-five of which I did not need in order to be at my optimal weight. I knew I was missing something important. But what? My life was in shambles, my health wrecked from the eating disorder, my marriage falling apart, and my business about to go under. I woke up one morning and couldn't get out of bed. I wanted nothing more than to be dead. I knew in that moment I had a choice to make. I could let the weight of life crush me or I could fix what was broken. The idea of digging myself out of the hole I was in was overwhelming, and yet I knew it was possible. Suicide would have been the easy way out. I knew I would have to pass through a dark night of the soul in order to heal but I also knew I could handle it. I resolved that day not only to live, but to thrive.

I hired dieticians. I went to twelve-step meetings. I had a therapist. I devoured spiritual books. I got a divorce. I sold my business. I took a solo multi-year road trip through Mexico where I learned to do body work and trained in big-wave surfing. I studied yoga in Bali. I became certified in clinical nutrition, personal training, reiki, and yoga. I learned a great deal and grew personally leaps and bounds. My happiness had improved dramatically, but the weight was still hanging around. I knew I was so close. There was just a small missing piece, but what?

Through my study, I learned that all physical imbalances, including illness, injury, and weight gain, are in response to a problem that starts long before our physical cells become damaged. In my case, weight gain was a symptom, and I was digging deep to find the root cause. Whenever we aren't treating the root cause, symptoms will worsen to the point that we are forced to pay attention. And that is exactly what happened to me. My body threw a new problem in the mix, a debilitating back injury which left me unable to walk, sit, or stand for more than five minutes at a time for about a year. Finally, my body had my attention. I knew healing would only come by putting the rest of life on hold (I had no choice in this case) and digging deep within. Because of the tools I had learned over the previous five years, I knew there was a major lesson in this injury, and I resolved to understand it. I spent the better part of my days in bed or lying on the beach meditating. For someone with clinical anxiety, this was excruciatingly difficult. But I knew that somehow this experience would be the key to overcoming whatever was still holding me back.

The answer came to me one morning in a flash. I can only describe it as a moment of grace, divine inspiration. The answer came to me in a banana.

I was very hungry as I headed to the beach in front of my house early one morning to do my meditation. I wanted to eat upon waking like I normally did, but something told me to do this meditation while fasting, an experiment I had never tried before. Strangely enough, after I dropped into a meditative state, my hunger was forgotten. After a few hours, I noticed a rumble in my stomach. I reached in my bag for the breakfast I had packed. I pulled out a banana. As I held it in my hand, I felt a rush of pleasure from the delightful texture of the peel. I held it for several minutes, just gazing at the color and enjoying the texture on my skin. It was mesmerizing. So mesmerizing that I forgot I was hungry. In fact, I *wasn't* hungry. The texture and the pleasure had somehow satiated me. Then I lifted the banana to my face and inhaled deeply. I was overwhelmed by its delightful smell, as if it was the first time I'd ever smelled a banana. It was too beautiful, the whole experience. That is when the code cracked for me. I realized in an instant that food was for pleasure as much as it was for fuel. I became acutely aware in that moment that I had been using food as my staple, and almost singular, source of comfort.

It was the moment when all that I had learned on my quest suddenly became synthesized and usable. Up until that point, I had been doing the work. I was learning what was available to me through books, professionals, support groups, travel, lifestyle changes, and certifications. Then I carved out the space to be still (or rather was forced into it). And when I was finally ready to understand the answers I so desperately sought, I saw them there in plain sight. Now my body's "check engine light" (weight) is turned off because I addressed the underlying problems. In the three months following that meditation, I lost twenty-five pounds without a second thought.

Body Alchemy is everything useful that I have learned about how to have a healthy body that you love without ever dieting again and none of the BS. I remember reading plenty of eating disorder books, telling me to take a warm bath or call a friend when I felt a binge coming on. I would laugh at these useless suggestions, intuitively knowing they were not going to solve the real problem. On the other hand, I remember friends and therapists suggesting, "You just need to be happy and learn to love yourself no matter what." To which I always wanted to reply, "Yeah, that sounds all well and good, but could you tell me *HOW*?" This book is the reply I was looking for and you will find it to be foundational in your journey as well.

Having a graduate degree in math, I love to take complex ideas and simplify them into simple and elegant formulas. I have done my best to throw out all of the woo-woo spiritual bypassing and include only what is absolutely essential to get you on the fast track to your happiest body ever so you can ditch the struggle with weight and move into your greatness NOW. Body Alchemy isn't a diet at all, but rather a powerful formula that delivers life changing results. Let's take a look at the overall formula before we discuss the specifics.

Diets fail at providing permanent weight loss because they don't treat the root cause of why a person wants to overeat in the first place. So it follows, treat the root cause and physical transformation will happen.

What happens when you get a cut? Your body closes it up without being asked. What happens when you get a cold? Your body heals up without medicine. What happens when your bladder gets full? Your body sends a signal to your brain and asks you to please urinate. Did you try to take your last breath or did your body breathe *you*? If you are a person with ovaries and you've made your own little person, how did you do that? Even the most brilliant and talented obstetrician cannot explain exactly how the female body makes humans, but we've been doing it since long before science was invented.

So if our bodies tell us to breathe when we need air, tell us to drink when we need water, tell us to urinate and defecate when we need to release waste products, then why are they asking us to overeat? The answer is one word: suffering.

Food is a temporary solution to suffering, both over and under eating. There is overwhelming scientific data showing how food changes brain chemistry. But you don't need to look any further than your own experience. Food makes us forget, calms us down, gives us something to do, cheers us up, and distracts us from all sorts of pain. We have associated eating with symptomatic relief from pain so much so that all pain starts to feel like hunger. Food is a fantastic pain killer. But like taking a painkiller for a broken arm, it's not going to solve the problem. So if suffering is the cause of overeating, then the solution logically follows: end suffering, end overeating. And in a world where we often feel completely out of control of our own suffering, we turn to food, the one thing we can control, to ease the pain. So how do we end suffering when we are simply not in control?

Obviously we can stop bad things from happening. Of course not. Loved ones die, wars rage, children starve. Pain is certainly inevitable! But suffering is optional. There is a well-known prayer that is repeated thousands of times a day in twelve-step meetings all over the world. The *Serenity Prayer* goes like this: "God, grant me the serenity to accept the things I cannot change, the courage to change the things that I can and the wisdom to know the difference." In this book, you will learn how to handle unavoidable pain with serenity, how to know when something painful needs to change, and how to make powerful changes when they are warranted. You will learn all of this in order to reduce, or even end, suffering. When this happens, the body falls in line with its natural rhythms once again and the cravings to eat more than what the body physically needs naturally disappear.

The formula appears to be very simple, and it is, but this oversimplification covers everything we must unpack in the pages to come. Now we must go about doing the work in order to get the result.

How to Read this Book

This book is divided into four parts. The first part focuses on ending the suffering caused by being out of alignment with our true purpose. This is the kind of suffering we can change by making external changes.

Part II is all about ending the suffering we cause ourselves by becoming too wrapped up in our thoughts. This is also suffering that we have the power to change by making internal changes.

The third part is a road map for cultivating serenity in the face of unavoidable pain. The aim of this section is to provide a framework and tools so that when pain presents itself, you will have the power to manage it without the addition of suffering.

Part IV of this book specifically addresses the body. This part of the book comes last for a reason. Skipping ahead is like trying to take a test before learning the material. You're bound for failure before you even start. Whatever is going on in your body is a symptom of something going on emotionally, mentally, and spiritually. That is why it is important that you read the first three sections of this book first and master the activities before moving on to address the body.

Throughout this book, I provide concrete tools to strengthen your awareness and put in the groundwork for true transformation. Just like a diet, I'll ask you to follow a few specific steps. But unlike a diet, they won't involve depriving yourself in any way. Actually, it will be the opposite.

I have only one rule I ask for you to follow throughout this entire process: *do what you want to do*. Nothing more, nothing less. Let every action you take be motivated by "want-power" not willpower. It is true that thoroughly completing every bit of homework, taking to heart every suggestion, and acting on this information immediately will provide the fastest and most powerful results, but, and this is a big but, the results will not be lasting. If you are simply not ready to make changes, or not enjoying the changes you are forcing yourself to make, eventually you will tire of doing them and go back to your old habits.

The approach I suggest instead is to do the homework as much as it brings you joy. Try out each suggestion and then let it go if it doesn't serve you. Perhaps you will pick up just one nugget of truth from this book that will then set you up to be ready for some encounter, workshop, or other delivery of transformational information down the road which would have otherwise fallen on deaf ears had you not read this book. Or perhaps you will pick up this book again in a year's time and find that you are now in a place where everything resonates with you and you are ready for big changes. You are ready when you are ready, not a moment before. So please don't guilt yourself into being an "A" student. Some people love homework assignments and thrive on being the high performer in the room. If that is you, then by all means have fun and do your best. But if you tend to be a back of the classroom kinda girl, don't worry; do what feels useful and leave the rest for another day.

I invite you to join our community at http://www.melanieezell.com/ where there is a discussion forum for each homework in this book. You will notice that each homework is numbered. On my website there is a corresponding thread for each number. This is a great way to get extra help, remain accountable and share insights with others.

Lastly, this book uses female nouns and pronouns. But Body Alchemy works equally for men or an individual who struggles with emotional and binge eating and is finally ready to ditch diets for good so they can find a body they love.

Part I Making External Changes

Chapter 1: Internal GPS

The first step to reduce suffering is to end self-inflicted pain. This means making bold changes to the things that can and need to be changed in our lives. The reality is that some pain is unavoidable, and we will cover that type of pain in Part III. But sometimes it is possible to remove the painful stimulus altogether, which is certainly preferable, but often takes great courage and commitment. In this chapter, we will look at the things in our lives that need to change and can be changed. I will present a framework for knowing if change needs to be made, how to make that change easily, and how to find more moments in your life where everything is flowing and painful stimuli are at a minimum. Although this might sound daunting, remember you have full permission to work at your own pace, doing what feels right when it feels right.

I like to think of a boardroom up in heaven. The label on the door says, "New Human Programming." In that room, there is a group of angels in charge of solving humanity's problems. They can see the whole picture from up there and they know exactly what needs to be done to move humanity forward in evolution. So they design each new baby to fulfill a critical role toward that end. But how will the baby know what she needs to do when the time comes to do it? How will she find herself in the right place at the right time? How will she learn the skills necessary in her lifetime in order to accomplish her mission? These angels do not override a human's free will. Instead, they give each new human a road map, like GPS. If they choose to follow the GPS, they will accomplish their mission. So what is this GPS? The desires of the heart. Each turn-by-turn direction sounds like a desire to do or say something. Unfortunately, each time an authority figure tells that child that she "shouldn't" do that, the volume on the GPS gets turned down a tiny bit. And by the time most children reach adulthood, the GPS is at such a low volume that they can't hear it at all. They find themselves staring at a restaurant menu, making a choice based not on the description of the food that sounds best, but on the calorie count next to the description. Worse yet, they are at that restaurant for a business meeting they don't want to be in, making money in a career that doesn't bring them joy to support an oversized mortgage in a city they never wanted to stay in.

Everything you need to know about how to live your best life was programmed into you from the very beginning. When we fail to live the life we were meant for, suffering is inevitable. By the time most of us reach adulthood, we have made many compromises with the world and given up much of our individuality in order to fit in. This inauthenticity is a recipe for comfort-seeking behaviors, such as overeating. The solution? Reclaim our personal power.

I distinguish hunger into two categories: lower case "h" hunger, and upper case "H" Hunger. Little h hunger is when your belly is rumbling, your blood sugar is getting low, and you need to eat some food to provide for the energetic needs of your body. Big H Hunger is everything else. It is the way we wished we looked in that dress, the man we thought we married who turned into someone else, the trip we never made time for, the fling we will never allow ourselves, the career we'd like to be building while we work as a cog in someone else's machine. Big H hunger is every moment of every day. Little h hunger strikes about three times a day for most people. But we've buried our Hungers so deep and heaped on the guilt and shame so high that we don't even admit to ourselves how badly we want to run. We want to bolt out of the cubicle, out of the relationship, out of the country. But we won't admit it. So instead we bolt into a bowl of caramel swirl ice cream. We bolt to our vibrators, our social media feeds, our online shopping apps. We bolt higher up the corporate ladder and deeper into our kids' sports and constant activities. Meanwhile, we grab a mocha Frappuccino and a candy bar disguised as a protein meal to replace all the energy consumed from living an inauthentic life. I know. I've lived it. And it doesn't have to stay that way.

The key is to trust our desires as much as we trust an urge to use the bathroom.

Chapter 2: You Are Not Flawed

The other day, I was talking to a friend about a problem he was having with his sons. It seemed every time the younger son was getting positive affirmations from the parents, the older son felt the need to steal the show. My friend exclaimed, "You see, he just has this flaw. He was born with no empathy!" I happen to know that this particular pregnancy for the older son wasn't wanted. It took my friend, the father, until the boy was almost two years old to even accept him and to show affection for him. Although he is certainly loved and cared for now, his parents remain very busy with their careers and one-on-one attention is still in short supply. "So you would rather believe that your child came to you flawed from the womb than that you, as a parent, have failed him?" I asked my friend.

Most of our parents loved us unconditionally but to children, punishment comes across as the removal of love. And rewards for good behavior further engrain the feeling of conditional love. Unintentionally, even the best parents may have made us believe we were flawed from birth. Here is the thing, many many people have a huge investment in making us feel like we are flawed. My friend, the father, has a religious belief system that teaches all people are fundamentally evil. We are born depraved. We are all "wretches" as the most famous Christian hymn puts it. I'm not convinced your local Paster wants you to feel like a big screw up but unfortunately that is how people, especially children, receive that message. I believe this is one of the most misunderstood doctrins in the Christian church. We were not born broken, we were born into brokenness. The difference is subtle but life changing. Even if you weren't raised in a religious tradition, the thinking still permeates our culture. Our parents disciplined us to get us to change our behavior, sending us the message that there was something wrong with us. Overworked teachers reinforced this thinking by sending unruly students to detention rather than seeking to understand why the student doesn't care to learn in the first place. Children raised on punishments and rewards are bound to grow into adulthood thinking that there is always improvement to be made and putting their trust into "experts" for guidance rather than looking inward. Can you see it? A diet is nothing more than another way to "be a good girl." Just follow these rules and you'll be accepted, rewarded, and liked. But dare to break the rules and you'll be a fat slob from whom Mom and Dad will withdraw their love.

And it's all a lie. Religion (opposed to spirituality and relationship with God), parents, political leaders, advertisers, and bosses all have the same motive for making us feel wrong. Because if we believe we are flawed, then we will put our trust into their hands and thereby acquiesce our power. My friend's son happens to be one powerful little boy, but his parents are creating a self-fulfilling prophecy.

You too are powerful. You have forgotten, but not entirely. And that is why you're holding this book. Because the part of you that feels most authentically like *you,* that part remembers. Some part of you wants to throw your fist up at diet culture, burn not just your bra but also the white picketed life you've responsibly built. A little piece of you wants to run off to live a life in the jungle. Even though you were raised in captivity, you know, deep down inside, you are a wild beast. And something about keeping your body in check with good-girl lists and rules seems both appealing and so wrong. The thing is, everything you need to know is already inside you. You already know every rule for how to live *your* unique best life. It is called intuition.

Even if you are morbidly obese and your weight is significantly affecting your health, even killing you, your hunger can still be trusted. Because your hunger is alerting you to the fact that you NEED something. You may have become confused about what it is that you need exactly and so food takes the place of a deep yearning for nourishment of another kind. But one thing is certain: cutting out the food is not going to heal you unless you replace it with the nourishment your body is truly craving. And this is the reason diets almost never work. They take away the food without providing an alternative source of nourishment.

This is why it is not just our desire for food that needs to be trusted, but rather ALL of the things we want, hope, and dream for. And this is why intuitive eating alone isn't enough. Because if we are depriving ourselves in other areas of our lives but we've removed food restrictions, then all the things we don't allow ourselves will show up on your plates.

Chapter 3: Desires Can Be Trusted

Another particularly soul crushing cultural presupposition we were handed in our developmental years is the idea that our desires are evil. Of course, if we were born sinful, or trained to be "good little girls," then at some point we had to sacrifice what we wanted for the sake of what someone else wanted from us. I see it in my toddler and my reactions to him all the time. He wants to throw things around the house to see how high they can go, pull everything off the shelf to see what is behind it, and express every emotion as loud and annoyingly as possible. I, of course, do not want any of those things. Conventional parenting says to use rewards and punishments to get him to "behave." The fact is there is nothing evil about his behavior. He is a curious toddler eager to learn. Getting into everything is how he does it. He isn't "naughty," he is a two-year-old. Punishment for doing what his instincts say to do would make him feel naughty and wrong.

The truth is that a little more attention from me, directing him into more appropriate learning activities, is really what he needs. We have been tamed, dear sisters. We went to schools that forced us to sit in neat rows for hours on end, preparing us to work in neat cubicles for even more hours. Then we took out loans so we could get more education so we could get good jobs so we could work long hours so we could pay back the loans. We've become circus tigers. We jump through hoops for rewards from people we could easily eat for a small snack. We have forgotten; we have been wild all along. But thank God for chocolate chip cookies. Ooey, gooey, thick, soft but slightly crunchy chocolate chip cookies. Because just when we think we can't possibly jump through one more flaming circus hoop, just when we think we might actually tear all those people to shreds—well that's when at last the kids are in bed and *The Bachelorette* is on and as long as you agree to play by the rules just one more day, you might as well reward yourself with a cookie… or four.

Here is the truth. You are wild. You were born that way. You were meant to be that way. And even though you've been domesticated, wild blood still flows in your veins. And until you release yourself from captivity and learn to survive in the wild on your own, you will continue to self-medicate with food, shopping, dating apps, or whatever makes you forget your wild beast the fastest.

Here is an important concept. You were born with a purpose. You came to Earth to do something. Each of us has. Steven Pressfield says it like this, "If you were meant to cure cancer or write a symphony or crack cold fusion and you don't do it, you not only hurt yourself, even destroy yourself, you hurt your children. You hurt me. You hurt the planet… Don't cheat us of your contributions… God created you with the sole purpose of nudging the entire human race one millimeter forward." From the beginning of time, as far back as science understands, the universe has been evolving, one millimeter at a time. Let's make a rough sketch of what that evolution has looked like:

There was once nothing but pure potential energy. Energy became heat, and there was a bang. Out of that heat, stars formed. Then raw elements were synthesized from within the stars. The elements came together to form atoms. The atoms came together to form molecules. The molecules came together to form cells. Then cells became organisms, and organisms became plants, animals, and humans. Okay, so apart from an interesting review of middle school science, why am I bringing this up? Because it is all going somewhere. All of *this* is moving forward. Each new step in the evolutionary trajectory is toward something more communal, more complex, more intelligent. And you have a critical mission within the process of it all. It is why you are here. The universe needs you to combine your unique talents and strengths with all of ours so that we can build something better. Some traditions call it your Dharma. You have a mission to accomplish while you are here. And you know who knows exactly and precisely what that mission is? You, specifically, your desires.

So how the heck do we release ourselves from self-imposed captivity back into the wild? How do we orient ourselves back to the purpose those angles designed us for? How do we turn up the volume on the GPS? How do we listen to our hearts again?

This journey begins like any other, with one terrifying step after another in an unknown direction. The first step is to trust that whatever you desire, no matter how depraved, messed up or out of the norm it may seem, it can be trusted. From here on out, there is no such thing as wants and needs. They are the same. If you want something, you need it. When you don't act on your desires, your body will find another way to satisfy that big "H" Hunger, normally by making you little "h" hungry. Often our desires seem terribly "naughty" and we are afraid to admit them, even to ourselves. Sometimes, even desires that lead down painful paths are exactly what we need to ultimately lead us to fulfilled lives. Let me explain.

I had the pleasure of meeting a relationship and sexuality coach. As a teen she was wildly sexual and quickly found a successful career as an exotic dancer at the age of 18. At the time, everyone around her judged her choices as being poor and assumed she would end up on a very painful path. Having no one to rely on but herself and not having good parental influence, she continued to do what she needed to make ends meet, not caring what anyone thought. The truth is, she did have some hard times and experienced a lot of pain as direct and indirect consequences of her choices. We all do. Later she became successful supporting and counselling new mothers, also having a strong love for women and children. The two careers seemed worlds apart. Now, two decades later, after many twists and turns, she helps couples with small children to have better relationships, including in the bedroom. She could not have been as effective without her firsthand knowledge. Now she is saving marriages; she is saving families. Every day by being true to herself, she moves evolution forward. This is what I want for you. Could there have been a less destructive or softer way for her? Who knows. But what we do know is that no matter what, as long as you keep seeking, you will find what you are looking for. No matter your path, it can be used for good. You haven't made any mistakes, you've just done the best you could with what you had.

In order to move into the person we were designed to be, we must rid ourselves of black and white thinking. Black and white thinking is a cognitive distortion. A cognitive distortion is a fancy word for a way we are programmed to think that isn't helpful. When one falls into the trap of black and while thinking, they apply labels, making one option entirely wrong and another entirely right. For example, "Sugar is bad." It is? What if you're at mile twenty in a marathon and your body has run out of glucose? What if you're a diabetic having a blood sugar crash? What if you're depressed and the idea of a chocolate chip cookie gets you out of bed and into the fresh air for a walk to the bakery? You get the idea. In the case of my friend above, many may have labelled her work as "bad" because it conflicted with their value system. It may have been bad for me, and there arguably may have been an easier way for her, but in the end it all worked out for her greatest good. Another more subtle way black and white thinking affects us is in thinking one instance generalizes to the whole. For example, "My boyfriend forgot my birthday; therefore, he doesn't love me." Or "I cheated on my diet; I might as well binge." Do you see where there is a whole lot of room for gray? I recently saw black and white thinking in a social media battle about professional sports and the inclusion of transgender people. The "open minded" side called someone who raised questions a "bigot." There was no room for gray. The black and white thinking goes, "If one does not accept this ruling about transgender inclusion as completely correct, they are a completely bad human." Black and white thinking is behind all hate crimes, labels, and acts of discrimination everywhere. When we start to wake up to our own tendencies to apply black and white judgments toward ourselves, we begin to open the world to a new way of thinking. That is why it is so critical at this time in history to do the work of internal healing. As the NPR show *New Dimensions Radio* puts it, "It is only through a change in human consciousness that the world will be transformed. The personal and the planetary are connected."

The problem with black and white thinking is that it often tries to override our internal GPS. We were raised to believe a certain thing is bad and so we avoid it, even though we desperately want to do it. Sexuality and self expression are big ones here. And so are our rules about what we should and should not eat. But whenever something is forbidden, it makes it more alluring. From here on out, whenever a little voice in the back of your head says, "Oh but I shouldn't," or "But I can't," recognize that for what it is, a cognitive distortion and ultimately a pathology. Question everything.

Time for a little bit of concrete practice with these abstract ideas. This homework is simple and powerful. Just turn up the volume on your GPS. Don't even worry about following the GPS right now. Just acknowledge it is there. It is time to start admitting to ourselves what we want and desire. If you feel like taking a chance and acting on your desires, you can. Just know that we have a little more to discuss on the topic of consequences. So for now, just listening is enough. Take time to write or say aloud or in your mind what you desire, no matter how "naughty" it might seem. Examples I've seen from clients are "I want to quit my job," "I want to get away from my partner for an extended vacation," "I want to eat cheese on everything," "I want to get Botox," "I want to stay home." And don't forget about the things you don't want. "I don't want to take out the trash," "I don't want to have sex."

This activity is especially illuminating when there is something you want that conflicts with your value system. This happens a lot with sexual thoughts and thoughts toward people we love. For example I might think, "I want to hit my child right now." Wow! When I bring light to that thought I am able to see that I have work to be done in the anger and patience departments. It is only by bringing light to our darkest corners that we can find healing. Most religious practise some kind of confession. Confession is the first step toward repentance. First confess, or admit to yourself, what you are struggling with.

Again, for *now,* until we talk about sitting with emotions and observing consequences, I don't advise acting on every desire. But there will be a time when you will be able to let loose without ruining your life, I promise! Happy wanting!

Chapter 4: Core Values

Each of us comes into existence with a unique personality. As I mentioned before, this personality was divinely and meticulously crafted to serve you in completing your highest good. Our personality, along with our upbringing and conditioning, form our "Core Values." Core values are a deeply ingrained (although changeable) operating system from which we make decisions big and small. For example, my husband's deepest core value involves recreation, while my deepest value involves growth. We both love to surf. When he surfs, it is about pure fun while I am often seeking out coaches and feedback, always trying to improve the way I surf. Neither approach is wrong. Recreation brings my husband joy while growth brings me joy.

We all make subconscious decisions based on our core values every day, from what to wear to how we keep the house. Again, for example, my husband would rather lie down in a messy house and read a fiction book while I would rather listen to a personal development book on audio while cleaning the house. Ironically, it is the bigger decisions where we tend to stray from our core values. Conditioning and a long list of "shoulds," cultural norms, and familial expectations leave us confused when it comes to decisions like where to live, what career to choose, and who to marry. Obviously, this sets us up for a very unsatisfying life. One day you find yourself in the middle of your workday saying, "Why am I doing any of this?" You've strayed too far from your true self and your heart knows it. But so much easier than admitting it is covering it up. Because it is way easier to eat pizza and drink beer than it is to quit your job, ditch your partner, and go back to school in your forties for the career you always wanted but never dared to try.

So the time has come to become intimately familiar with what makes you tick. What are your core values? There are no "wrong" core values. One of my core values used to be "attention," specifically attention from men. As I was able to admit this to myself and allow myself to go off seeking (and finding) attention, it lost a great deal of its allure. This value still plays a part in my current value system, but it has changed from "attention" to "audience," specifically an audience of people to whom I can be of service. But it was only through exploring the value of attention that I was able to grow and mature. One day, with more maturity, this value may drop away altogether and that will be fine too.

There are two activities you will need to complete in order to discover your core values. Please take your time and complete these when you are ready. Make sure you have space and time to yourself where you won't be interrupted. Again, as with all suggestions and homework, do what feels joyful and useful. Do as much as feels fun and when you don't feel like doing it anymore, stop.

Homework 1: *A Few of My Favorite Things*

For this activity you will need:
- Sticky notes (or little pieces of paper + tape)
- A large blank wall or empty counter/table
- Timer/cellphone on focus mode with timer
- Pen

1. Grab your sticky notes. Set a timer for five minutes.
2. Start writing down your favorite things in life, one item on each sticky note. Ex: Time with my son, surfing, feeling cute, helping women find their purpose, etc.
3. Don't restrict yourself, just get as much out there as you can.
4. After the time is up, start organizing the sticky notes into groups. For example, I might put surfing, sunsets, jogging, yoga, and smoothies into one group. In another group I might put writing, public speaking, helping women, photo editing, and social media into another group.

5. Try to have four to five groups. If you have more, combine them or toss out things that seem the least valuable.
6. Give each group a label. For the examples above I might choose FITNESS and CONTRIBUTION, respectively.
7. Next rank these groups in order of importance. These are your core values.

Homework 2: *Make a List*

1. From the list below, choose and write down every value that resonates deeply with you. There will be lots that resonate a little but pick the ones that are most powerful. Work quickly, don't overthink it.
2. Group similar words together into about five groupings. You can use five colored highlighters or just re-write the values into five new groupings. For example: Wealth, security, free-time, flexibility, and influence could make one category. A second could be: kindness, inclusion, gratitude, friendship, community.
3. Choose a label for each group. It could be a word from within the group or a label that makes sense. For the above examples the label for the first group could be "Financial Success" while the label for the second group might be "Friendship."
4. Now add a verb to each label to make it actionable. Such as "Become financially successful" and "Cultivate friendships."
5. Write your core values in order of importance.

Abundance	Dedication	Kindness	Professionalism
Acceptance	Dependability	Knowledge	Punctuality
Accountability	Diversity	Leadership	Relationships
Achievement	Empathy	Learning	Reliability
Adventure	Encouragement	Love	Resilience
Advocacy	Enthusiasm	Loyalty	Resourcefulness
Ambition	Ethics	Making a	Responsibility
Appreciation	Excellence	Difference	Responsiveness
Attractiveness	Expressiveness	Mindfulness	Security
Autonomy	Fairness	Motivation	Self-Control
Balance	Family	Optimism	Selflessness
Being the	Friendships	Open-	Simplicity
Best	Flexibility	Mindedness	Stability
Benevolence	Freedom	Originality	Success
Boldness	Fun	Passion	Teamwork
Brilliance	Generosity	Performance	Thankfulness
Calmness	Grace	Personal	Thoughtfulness
Caring	Growth	Development	Traditionalism
Challenge	Flexibility	Proactive	Trustworthiness
Charity	Happiness	Professionalism	Understanding
Cheerfulness	Health	Quality	Uniqueness
Cleverness	Honesty	Recognition	Usefulness
Community	Humility	Risk Taking	Versatility
Commitment	Humor	Safety	Vision
Compassion	Inclusiveness	Security	Warmth
Cooperation	Independence	Service	Wealth
Collaboration	Individuality	Spirituality	Well-Being
Consistency	Innovation	Stability	Wisdom
Contribution	Inspiration	Peace	Zeal
Creativity	Intelligence	Perfection	
Credibility	Intuition	Playfulness	
Curiosity	Joy	Popularity	
Daring		Power	
Decisiveness		Preparedness	
		Proactivity	

Adapted from taproot.com

Once you've completed both activities, synthesize your results into one list with four to six core values. Write them in a way that feels good to you, either as full sentences, verb + value or as single words. Take a photo of this list or write it in a note on your phone so you can refer to it whenever you are faced with a tough choice.

Chapter 5: Consciousness

Before we can go forward to act on our desires and core values, we must first become conscious of what is going on in the mind. While acting on desires and values with consciousness will lead toward the end of suffering, acting on desires and values without consciousness is a sure path toward suffering. So let's look at the difference here.

Consciousness is a buzzword these days. It's thrown around a lot, to the point that it sounds a bit like jargon. So let me be clear what I mean by consciousness. The clearest definition I can give is an experiential one. So let's do a brief exercise. Wherever you are right now, take a deep breath. Close your eyes if it is safe to do so. Feel your feet or butt pressing into whatever is beneath you. In a moment I will ask you to stop reading and do your best to think about nothing. Since this is pretty much impossible, thoughts will come up quite quickly. Instead of dwelling on them just try to notice the content of the thought. For example, "Oh, I'm thinking about the way my back is aching," or "Oh, I am thinking about what I need to get done after I read this book." Just make a quick assessment of the thought and then go back to thinking about nothing. Do this for the first three thoughts that come up. Ready, go!

Okay. That is it. That is *what,* you might ask. That is consciousness. The moments when we are aware of our thoughts but not identified with them. In other words, we know that we are thinking but we are not necessarily acting on the thoughts or even believing the validity of the thoughts. You might think that you are always aware of your thoughts, but the truth is that almost no one is aware of their thoughts all the time. Research shows that our subconscious runs about 90-95% of our programming. Most of us are unaware that we are even thinking most of the time. We have imagined conversations in our heads. We think about the way people should be acting. We make judgments. We feel sad about the past. We worry about the future. We try to decide what we should say next. To be conscious is to be in the present moment. If you want to know if you are unconscious, simply ask, *"Are my thoughts about the here and now or are they in the past or future or an imaginary place other than here?"*

Let's try another exercise. Once you finish reading these words, scan your body for areas of tension and pain. Just notice what feels off today. Ready? Go!

Again, that is consciousness. It is all about what you are noticing here and now. It is that simple, all of your thoughts were in the present moment and were regarding sensations happening now and locally. And I bet you were surprised to find a lot of areas of tension that you've just been living with. Most of us don't even know we are in pain until we are out of it!

But, did you have any thoughts like, "I should be stretching more," or "How can I fix this?" Were you aware that you were having those thoughts before I asked? If not, then those were unconscious thoughts. We are NEVER going to stop the thoughts from coming. The idea is to *notice* the thinking. And then decide if we want to keep that thought or toss it out. So if you thought, "I should be stretching more," let's take a look at that. Do you have time to make stretching a priority? Would it enhance the quality of your life if you prioritized stretching? Would you enjoy doing it? Based on the answers to those questions, is the thought "I should be stretching more" a thought you want to keep? If so, make a plan for when you will fit stretching into your day. Then let all thoughts of stretching go. Now that you have a plan, move on. When the time is right to enact your plan, do so. And if you decide stretching really isn't worth it, notice that this thought, "I should be stretching more" really isn't useful. The next time it comes up, if you are conscious and aware that you are thinking that thought again, then you can have a little laugh. "Oh my silly repetitive brain. I don't need that thought anymore, thanks anyway!" And then you can move on guilt free.

So consciousness is being aware of your thoughts by bringing your attention to the here and now. And what does this have to do with weight, bodies, and eating? EVERYTHING! Because it takes a thought to move our arms and legs to the pantry. Typically an unconscious thought. It goes like this: It's been a long day, but the kids are finally in bed. Before you know it, you're holding a package of Oreos and scrolling social media. But what happens between the kids are asleep and Oreos? A lot! The unconscious thoughts are flying through your head at warp speed. "Oh mygoodness! I'm exhausted. This day was a doozy! I can't believe it took forty minutes to get my daughter to stay in bed. I thought we were through this stage. This is the only 'me' time I get all day. If we have to go back to sleep training, I'm going to lose so much of my free time again. And now I'm too beat to do the yoga video I was going to do. Screw it. Maybe tomorrow. Today is just a bad day and I'll just enjoy something sweet to take my mind off this whole thing. I totally deserve a reward after all that. I worked my ass off today and nobody but myself is going to appreciate it. I think we still have left over pizza. Should I eat that? No. Too many calories. I'll just have one Oreo. Where is my phone? Geeze, seventeen emails. Nope, I'm too tired tonight. [Clicks social media app]. Oh this couch feels good..." Forty-five minutes later… "Oh shoot it's getting late and I still haven't paid those bills. OMG, I just ate the last Oreo!"

So in the example above there are three types of consciousness going on. There is the unconscious time, the time between when the daughter goes to sleep, and when the mom drops onto the couch with a package of Oreos. She is thinking but is unaware that she is thinking. Then there is the period of time, forty-five minutes, of scrolling and eating. In that time she is below consciousness. There is no real thinking going on. She is mostly unaware, blissfully unaware. Then there is the moment of consciousness. When she realizes the time and how much she has just eaten. In that moment she is squarely in the here and now. So the three types of consciousness are:

1. Below consciousness - Doing a compulsive behavior to drop below the level of thinking such as watching TV, shopping, scrolling social media or eating. Note that all of these behaviors certainly can be done consciously but are often done in a below conscious state.
2. Unconscious - In this state the mind is doing a lot of thinking but one is unaware they are having thoughts at all. Emotions and behaviors are being controlled by these thoughts without realization.
3. Consciousness - The state in which one is aware of their thoughts. Also an understanding that our true nature is the observer of thoughts rather than the thoughts themselves.

The important thing to understand here is that time spent in unconsciousness leads to suffering. For example, I may notice that my husband has not cleaned up the kitchen after dinner. This is a simple conscious thought. It is not a positive or negative thought, but rather an observation. It is completely neutral. I may then have a thought, "My husband doesn't appreciate the effort I put into making dinner." If I am unaware that I've had this thought then I may go about the kitchen cleaning plates and wiping counters with resentment and bitterness, continuing to feel disrespected and unappreciated. I may even add more to the story. "He never pitches in his fair share. I'm so overworked already and there he is looking at his phone. My life is totally unfair. He doesn't even love me." If I am unaware that my mind is inventing a very large story I will experience anger, frustration, stress, and a host of unpleasant emotions. And what do we do with unpleasant emotions? Well, we look for a way of making them go away. So I might try talking to my husband. He may feel defensive since I'm coming at him in anger, and he may withdraw in silence or retaliate in anger. In this case I'll need another solution to this new suffering. This is when many of us turn to the "below consciousness" behaviors because we just need something to make the thinking shut off. This is when a lot of us eat when we don't really need food for physical reasons. Which in turn will lead to more suffering (in the long run) and more below consciousness time and the cycle gets worse.

So the progression can be summed up like this: Unconscious thinking -> Suffering -> Below conscious behaviors -> More suffering.

So you might be thinking, "But you cooked! He needs to clean the kitchen already!" Okay. Let's take a look at this another way. I notice my husband hasn't cleaned the kitchen after dinner. The unconscious thought arises, "My husband doesn't appreciate the effort I put into making dinner." BUT I notice this thought. I evaluate it. *Does* my husband appreciate my effort? The only way to know that is to ask him. I can also ask him why he didn't clean the kitchen. I can consciously notice the unconscious assumption I just made. "I have an assumption that if I cook my husband will clean." I can express this assumption to my husband and ask him if he shares the same assumption. If he agrees I can ask him why he didn't clean. He may have been eager to get a jump start on tomorrow's emails. He may have thought he cleaned when in reality, his definition of clean and mine are different. Perhaps he simply doesn't appreciate my effort. In that case I can discontinue cooking for him because it doesn't really matter to him if I cook or not. In all of the above cases I eliminate the suffering that comes from having an unconscious thought if I can simply be aware of the thought and all of the thoughts and actions that come from it. Now I have more energy in my evening for doing things I need to do or enjoy doing. The next day I am better prepared to have an easier day. Life is now slightly less stressful. I am not being triggered to look for comfort in the form of food because I'm not uncomfortable in the first place.

In this case the progression looks like this: Unconscious thought -> consciousness intervenes -> Suffering avoided -> Progress made

So there are two opposite cycles we can enter into, the upward and the downward. And it is all a matter of applying consciousness. Now let's be very clear here. This isn't easy. Simple, yes, easy no. It takes practice, like anything worth doing. So that is where this homework is going to be very important!

Homework 3:
Mindfulness meditation
If possible, carve out a few minutes (between three and twenty) to sit in a quiet place with no distractions. The goal is to notice your thoughts. Note that the goal is not to eliminate thoughts, but rather to catch yourself while having them. If you don't have time or would like extra practice, you can do this while in the midst of any other menial task. Practice noticing your thoughts while washing dishes, riding in a car, cooking, etc. Continue this homework as often as possible.

Chapter 6: Conscious Allowing

So now that we know what consciousness is, let's marry consciousness with allowing. Allowing means to give permission to do something. From here on out you have permission to do anything and everything. Want to eat twenty-five chocolate chip cookies? Go buck wild! Want to quit your job? Go streaking through the halls of your office my friend! Okay, maybe not. Let me explain.

What I'm suggesting is that you allow yourself to consider anything and everything as a possible valid option. This is where hidden urges and cravings are completely allowed to come to the surface. Behind every urge, including the urge to eat what we don't physically need, is a reason, a perfectly valid reason. We might not physically need the food but some part of us needs nourishment. So urges should never be ignored. However, they may or may not need to be expressed in the way that feels most urgent. For example, whenever I am sleep deprived or overly stressed, I crave caffeine and sugar. While caffeine and sugar will help get me through the day, they will not solve the problem. What I *need* is rest and recreation. By sensing the urge for caffeine and sugar I can open myself to consciousness. "I want a caramel latte and it's four pm. This isn't quite normal for me. How would that make me feel? Awake. But it might keep me up late and it is definitely going to cause a crash later. What was I thinking about just before the craving hit? Oh, my dinner meeting. I hate dinner meetings. It makes for such a long day, and I have to skip my yoga class. Okay, I'm going to have that latte, but this is the last dinner meeting I'm agreeing to." In this way I have allowed myself what I wanted but also addressed the root cause of why I had the desire in the first place.

Let's say you have an urge to open up the shopping app on your phone and buy an item that feels like a bit of an indulgence. Consider doing it. Mentally walk yourself through the process. What will it feel like to look for the item, to read the reviews, then add the item to your cart? How will you feel the minute you hit "confirm purchase"? How will you feel when the item arrives in the mail? How will you feel when you check your credit card statement weeks later? How will you feel three months from now when the item is taking up space in your house? After all these considerations do you still want the item? Okay, go for it! And then notice every step. Notice the feeling of reading the reviews, adding it to your cart, paying the credit card bill, storing the item, etc. Notice every little bit of it. The next time you find yourself in a similar situation you will have heaps of mental data to draw on when making your decision. If you have any tendency toward compulsive shopping, simply bringing this kind of awareness will absolutely change your life. I've been in a fitting room, knee deep in clothing, only to be shaken awake with a moment of consciousness. The thought, "None of this will make my life any better right now" would hit me and I'd walk out of the store empty handed and happy.

Now let's take a look at a desire with big consequences, like leaving a relationship, moving houses, or quitting a job. Once again, if you are feeling an urge, there is a reason, a perfectly valid reason, for what you are feeling. You need to find that reason. But you can't find the reason if you don't admit to yourself that the desire is there, and that it is valid. You might start thinking through the consequences of, say, leaving a job, and realize that you'd simply have to get another job, and you'd still be unhappy because you won't be spending time with your family. It dawns on you, it isn't the job you hate but the time away from your family. Then you have options, downsize and work less, find remote work, cut back on your hours and save money on private school by homeschooling and spending more time with the kids, etc. Perhaps you really do dislike the work you are doing. Once you admit this, you can start making small steps that add up to big changes. We will discuss this in chapter nine.

And, of course, for every desire you decide to act on, you do so with 100% mindfulness. You notice how you feel before, during, after, and in the distant future as well. This is the way real and lasting change happens. It is very easy to avoid peanut butter if you have a peanut allergy, right? The idea here is the same: over time you will notice if something is making you feel bad and you won't want it in your life any more. No willpower involved.

Homework 4:
Mindful "below consciousness" behaviors

The next time you want to do a behavior that is typically "below consciousness" such as scrolling social media or eating when you know you don't physically need it, go ahead and do it! If you feel an unstoppable craving such as the urge to binge, this is the perfect time to do this homework! Just do it with incredible consciousness. What does the food feel like in your hand? What happens to your saliva as you consider taking a bite? Or maybe it is the urge to drop on the couch and scroll through social media. How do the colors on the screen make your eyes feel? Can you feel the radiation from the phone tingling in your hand? How many tiny details of the entire process can you notice? Then when it is all over, how do you feel? Do you feel better, worse, or the same? Are you more tired? Does your soul feel more alive? Continue to be hyper aware even into the next day to see if you can continue to feel the aftereffects of this behavior. Please note there should be NO GUILT in this activity. The idea is to bring things into your awareness to see if they enhance your life or not. And if you do feel guilt, notice it, have a little laugh, and move on.

Chapter 7: Mapping Yes and No

One of the biggest avoidable causes of suffering in life is saying yes when we would rather not and saying no when you really wanted to say yes. As we talked about, our desires inform our purpose. If we don't listen to our desires, it is like ignoring a GPS. The trajectory of our lives will be off kilter. We will always feel like *I know I was put here to do something, but this is definitely not it.* And that feeling of being off course will result in great suffering. Feeling like we are on the wrong path but not being sure how to find the right one will inevitably lead to behaviors that make us forget our pain, like dropping below consciousness. The only way to course correct is to start hearing and following our desires. Most of us don't even notice when we ignore our desires until it's too late, and the suffering is already happening.

I did it this morning. I haven't been feeling well recently. My brother is staying here to help me. My son had made a mess, and I was in the process of getting the vacuum out to clean it. My brother looked up from his work on his computer. "Mel, do you want me to do that?" I can see now that I had a super-fast unconscious conversation with myself that happened in a split second inside my brain. It went like this, "I would love to sit on my butt right now and let someone else deal with this. But my brother is busy working, and I don't want to interrupt him. My husband is over there reading a book. Why can't he do it? But I don't want to bother him while he's resting. Plus, I really am capable of doing this. It will be a little tiring but nothing I can't handle." Of course the whole point of my brother being here is so that I can avoid overly exerting myself and my husband can get a break. I quickly respond, "No, I got it!" Saying yes or no and meaning it takes a lot of practice and I'm still working on it! The first step, just like with emotional regulation, is to consciously spot the unconscious thoughts that have us saying the opposite of what we really want. This is going to take practice, and as I mentioned, I'm still working on it. We have been mixing up yes and no since early childhood when we first learned the meaning of the word "polite." But don't worry. Like anything, with practice it gets easier and easier.

We must get really familiar with the feeling of yes and no in the body. Yes and no have distinguishable signatures in the body which can be quickly read if we know how to do it. So let's take a minute right now to read them. Consider the following situation. You've just been asked if you want a $5000 gift card to your favorite clothing store! You've been feeling really good in your body recently and you need some new clothes. All you have to do is accept the gift card, no strings attached. Do you want it? Check in with your body. What sensations are you feeling? Are they moving? How would you describe them? Do they have colors or sounds? Where are they located? Assuming you answered, "ABSOLUTELY YES!" to the gift card, this is the signature of "yes" in your body. For me it is a brightness and widening of my eyes, an urge to smile, a tingling in my genitals, a lifting in my diaphragm, a widening of the rib cage.

Now let's take a look at another situation. An acquaintance from grade school whom you haven't spoken to in years has just sent you a message on social media. She and her family of six will be visiting your area soon for a vacation. She wants to stay at your house for ten days. What do you think? Check in with your body. Once again, map the sensations: where they are, what they feel and look like, and how they are moving. Assuming your answer was, "ABSOLUTELY NO," this is your map of "no" in your body. For me, this is a sinking in the pit of my stomach, the energy draining from my face, and a constriction in my throat. I recognized this feeling while I was vacuuming this morning and immediately noticed I was doing something I didn't want to be doing. It was recently enough (within minutes) so I was able to quickly bring up the unconscious chain of logic that had led me to the point of doing something I didn't want to be doing at all.

It isn't always clear at first if we want or do not want to do something. Often there are compelling reasons for both sides. But the heart knows what is best for you and has an opinion. Here are a couple of ways of extracting the opinions of the heart when in doubt.

1. Getting still. When in doubt take a few deep breaths. Sit down and close your eyes if you can. Picture yourself doing the thing. See how your body responds. Is it the yes signature, the no signature or something else? Now picture yourself not doing the thing. Again search for yes and no in your body's subtle reactions. Try not to overthink this. Just see how your body responds. Give yourself permission to hear what your heart wants and not necessarily act on it. Sometimes it is much easier to admit what your heart wants if you remove the pressure of obeying. Even just hearing the desires is a great place to start.

2. Muscle testing. Muscle testing is a way of visually noticing yes and no in your body. It's a bit more concrete than just feeling sensations. For this you will use your fingers to make the "Perfect" or "Okay" sign by making a loop with your index finger and thumb. Take the index finger of the other hand and put it inside the loop. With the loop hand try your best not to be broken and with the free index finger try your best to break through the loop. So each hand has a different goal. This is your reference. Notice how strong you are. It is probably impossible to break the loop. Now think about something that upsets you, stresses you out, or something you definitely don't want to do. With that in mind, try to break the loop. It will easily break. So that is your reference for something to be avoided. When you have a decision to make and you're not sure what your heart is telling you, make the loop, think of the situation, and see if it breaks. For example: Should you take a trip this summer to visit family, or should you stay home and save money? Consider staying home. Picture yourself going to work. Picture yourself on rent day

and try to feel those feelings knowing you've worked hard all month. Does the loop easily break or hold firm? Then picture the room you would stay in when visiting family. Picture the things you would be doing with them. Also picture yourself on rent day and try to feel those feelings. Now test the loop. What happens?

Muscle testing is a very useful way to see if your herbs and supplements are helpful to your body. Sit on a chair, put the bottle in your lap and try to break your loop. If it doesn't break, this is a beneficial herb. If it breaks, consider discontinuing its use. (Obviously you will need to talk to a doctor if this is prescription medication.)

3. Pendulum. Pendulums are nothing mystical or witchy. When you hold a pendulum out in front of you and ask it a question, it is not the pendulum that moves on its own, it is your arm that is moving it. But your arm is responding to your subconsciousness. Here is what I mean. Grab a necklace with a heavy pendant or tie a rock to the end of a string. This will serve as your pendulum. Hold it out at arm's length in front of you. Ask a simple "yes" question such as, "Is my name [your name]? Then let the pendulum swing. It will either swing left and right, away from you and back, or in a circle. Note how it swings. This is your "yes." Then ask a "no" question. "Do I have blonde hair?" (If you are a brunette.) The pendulum will swing the opposite way. This is your no. Now go ahead and ask your question. "Do I want to stay with my family this summer?" Be sure to picture yourself doing the thing you are asking about. The pendulum will start swinging yes or no and you will have your answer. If you want to believe the pendulum holds magical powers, feel free. But the reality is that nothing unscientific or woo-woo is going on here. You are simply allowing your own emotional response to take physical and visual form.

Homework 5:

Map yes and no in your body with simple questions which you already know the answers to.

Practice with muscle testing and the pendulum as well, using simple questions to which you already are certain of the answers. Once you feel comfortable try using your favorite of the three techniques on more ambiguous questions.

Now begin to use these three techniques with food choices. If you aren't sure what you want to eat, consider your options. With each option imagine yourself eating it. Then practice one of the three techniques to see how your body responds. If possible, you might even put the food in your lap (like a package of chips or an apple) and see how your body responds when the substance is within your energy field.

Chapter 8: Cornerstone Shifts

Knowing what you want is one thing, but acting on it is something else entirely. Have you ever stayed in a relationship, job, or living situation for much longer than you wanted to because you were afraid of ending it? Did the misery increase the longer you stayed? Did you feel huge relief soon after making the split? However big the discrepancy between your desires and actions will be the size of your suffering. Shortening this gap is essential if we are ever going to end the cravings to cover suffering with food or other unhelpful substances. Those of us who have been living under a long list of cultural and familial "shoulds" for our entire life have strayed so far from our desires that we have had to repress them entirely. Admitting to them is extremely painful because the idea of how much has to change is terrifying.

Don't be surprised if you discover this process challenging. Waking up one day and letting yourself say aloud, "I don't like the career I've invested a decade into," is one of the scariest things you can do. Because knowing what you don't want and doing it anyway is going to make life very difficult indeed, so it is easier not to admit to it at all. Which again, is why so many people are using food and other substances. Because even if they can admit they are miserable, they are too afraid to change. Covering that suffering with food is much easier than addressing it, even if it is killing them.

When you feel a big fat "no" inside your body and yet say "yes" anyway, it is important that you don't beat yourself up. Saying what you mean is going to take some practice so give yourself time. If you just can't get yourself to speak your truth don't worry about it. We are all a work in progress. Instead do the thing you don't want to do but do it mindfully the entire time, before, during, and after. Experience any discomfort that results. Don't run from the pain by doing a below consciousness behavior. Sit with the feeling in your body as much as possible. In the same way a child who touches a hot stove learns to stay far away in the future, by becoming hyper aware of how the choice to act incongruently with our truth feels, we will find it much easier to make a better choice next time. If you cannot or are not yet willing to say no and follow through, then see if you can change at least some part of the situation for next time.

For example, a client of mine, Julie, had a friend who had become very negative in everything she preferred to talk about. The friend never really wanted to do anything about her problems, she just wanted to complain, and she would always try to get Julie to agree with her about how awful it all was. It came to the point that Julie dreaded spending time with her friend. But they lived in the same neighborhood and the friend kept showing up at Julie's house and chatting her ear off about all her problems. She wanted so badly to tell her to leave but she couldn't bring herself to do it. She wasn't able to fully speak her truth. Instead, she simply stopped giving advice and empathy. She just listened and occasionally nodded. When the friend finished talking, Julie knew she wanted her to say how awful her problems were, but Julie was just honest and said something like, "None of this seems all that upsetting to me like it does to you right now." And then Julie would quiet down and let her friend rage on some more. After a few cycles of this the friend made an excuse and left. It still took more of her time than Julie really wanted to give her friend but at least she got the point. After this happened a few times, she quit showing up. A couple of years later they reconnected when the friend was in a better head space, and they resumed their friendship with no hard feelings.

This example shows how, even though Julie wasn't able to tell her friend directly that she would not tolerate her negativity, she could still find a way to avoid getting drawn into the drama of it all. The idea is to take small steps that have powerful trickle-down results. I am not going to suggest here that you make radical changes that seem really hard and terrify you. At least, not all at once. Of course, you are welcome to do so if you know in your heart it is time. But I don't want you doing anything that you aren't ready for. There is a simple and powerful way to soften the blow of making huge life-changing decisions: cornerstone shifts.

A cornerstone shift is one small change that has a powerful trickle-down result. I will illustrate this with a personal story. During one of the hardest times of my life, when I was most miserably stuck in my eating disorder, I desperately wanted to get better. I was working seventy–to-eighty-hour weeks. I was separated from my then-husband and considering divorce. My health was suffering, and I was extremely unhappy. My new business was struggling, and money was tighter than ever. I looked around my home one day and noticed piles of laundry and grime building up everywhere. I hadn't showered in four days. A week's worth of dishes were stacked in my sink. I realized, even if I didn't change anything else, I at least needed to take better care of myself. I decided I would make one easy change at a time. I resolved that no matter how stressful and jam packed my day, that I would drink at least eight cups of water per day. I didn't know it at the time, but this was my cornerstone shift.

The next morning I woke up to an empty water filter pitcher and a pile of dishes so high that I couldn't get the pitcher under the faucet to refill it. (Where I lived, no one drinks straight from the tap.) I was rushing out the door to meet my 6 am client and didn't have time to deal with it. I left my empty water bottle on the counter. That evening I got home late and didn't have the strength to do my dishes. I made a quick dinner and added more to the dish pile before going to bed. The next morning I had the same problem with no clean water to drink. The following evening I stayed up later than normal to do my dishes and clean the disgusting kitchen. I made it a priority even though I was tired. The following morning was brutal. I realized that 5 am wake ups were not working for me. I've never been a morning person. Something needed to go if I was going to be able to maintain a reasonable personal hygiene standard. It would have to be my 6 am client. I was scared because this was actually my best client and a significant portion of my income, which was already tight. I knew that if I gave up this client, I would not have enough income to cover my bills, which I had already whittled down to the point where there was nothing left to cut back on. I trusted that I would find a way. The extra time in my day allowed me to get a little extra sleep, maintain a (somewhat) clean house, do laundry weekly, shower daily, and of course fill my water bottle.

These new changes felt so good. I knew I wasn't willing to go back. But when it came time to pay bills, I was short. I wrote a check from my business account to my personal account to cover the difference. This went on for a few months. But eventually it caught up to me. My business was within a couple of months of going under. One day I had a meeting with a professional business coach. He asked me a lot of questions about overhead and my business model. He sat and thought for a couple of long minutes. Finally he broke the silence with words I will never forget. "Nope, doesn't work. Get out." A powerful and familiar feeling washed over me: relief. I wasn't disappointed, sad, combative, or anything of the sort. I was relieved. I had been wanting to call it quits on my business for a long time but up until that moment I hadn't been able to admit that to myself. When I heard those words and felt that feeling I knew I had been hiding my true desires from myself. Within a few months I had a buyer for my business, my divorce papers were signed, my bags were packed, and I set off on a transformational solo road trip down the Pacific coast of Mexico. I never came back to my life in that city. The job was gone, the husband was gone, and the old me was gone. My life changed in a massive way. But it started from a commitment to drink more water.

If I had woken up one day and decided to quit my life and drive to Mexico, it would have been an extremely difficult decision to follow through on. Even though that is what needed to happen, it happened naturally. And every step of the way was something I wanted to do, couldn't wait to do. There was no willpower involved. Want-power was my never-ending spring.

Your life may not be in shambles. You may not need to change much. Or you might need to change everything. You might have no idea what needs to change. But you don't have to have that figured out at all. All you need is to wake up each day and make small choices based on what you know you want and need *today*. In the above example all I knew was that I needed to take better care of myself. Some cornerstone shifts I've seen are: asking a partner to take on an additional hour of parenting time each day, committing to a weekly therapy session, purging items from the house in a big cleaning and committing to discarding an item every time a new item is brought home, cooking at home on weeknights, and many more. My favorite cornerstone shift, and the one I will suggest you begin with, is a morning (or evening) routine.

Routines are incredibly useful when our life feels chaotic. Something to hold onto each morning, no matter what the day brings, serves as a powerful anchor. I suggest a morning routine that includes the following.

- Something for the body (movement)
- Something for the mind (journaling, gratitude lists)
- Something for the soul (meditation, prayer, breathwork)

I suggest finding at least twenty minutes to do this. Here is how I suggest breaking it down:

Body: At least ten minutes. This could be yoga, body weight exercises, walking, tai chi, at home gym workout, workout video, etc. Whatever you *like*. It doesn't have to be strenuous. The main thing is that it feels good in your body. We will discuss exercise more in depth later. For now, just find a way of moving your body for ten continuous minutes that is enjoyable for you.

Mind: At least five minutes. Get your thoughts moving in a positive direction. Take a moment to write down goals for the day, things you are grateful for, any suppressed anxieties, positive affirmations, or visualizations of things you are manifesting. If you don't like to write, that is fine. Just find a few minutes to think through some of the above items and whisper your thoughts softly to yourself.

Soul: At least five minutes. This is a great time to practice noticing your thoughts. You can also pray or read a religious text such as the Bible if you have a religious practice or find that helpful. You could pick a breathing technique and try to stick to it for five minutes. The point is to connect to a deeper place, beyond thoughts. If you don't know where to start, there are many free meditations and breathing practices on the internet easily accessible with a quick search.

Twenty minutes is a huge ask, and at the same time is such a short amount of time. To be honest, I struggled with my morning routine once I became a mom. My son wakes up really early and immediately demands all of my attention. Yes, I could wake up earlier, but I don't want to. It is really hard to do that, and it takes a lot of willpower. So I gave up my morning practice. But I missed it so much that I adjusted it slightly and turned it into something I did after my son was in bed. But I was skipping it many nights because I was often very tired. I could feel myself a bit more frazzled and easily upset in general. I knew I desperately needed the precious time to myself. I have had very poor sleep since my son was born and really didn't want to give up his nap time for my own rest either. But I noticed I only needed a thirty-minute nap while my son slept almost ninety minutes. Since my husband was normally home when my son napped, I started getting up after I felt rested and heading to the beach for an hour of exercise, journaling, and meditation. I can't tell you how wonderful this felt after being away from it for some time. And then something amazing happened. Because I was often not back right when my son woke up, my husband started taking my son out for a bike ride. I would come home to a quiet house and have time to work or complete chores. The resentment I had toward my husband for having more free time than me started to drain and life got just a little easier. Once again, a cornerstone shift. Giving myself permission to be flexible is the entire reason I was still able to have any type of routine at all in the craziness that is new mom life. But I feel the withdrawal every time I drift away from this important time and that is what keeps me coming back to it. Once again, want-power over willpower!

Homework 6:

Develop a routine as laid out above. Try to implement the routine in the morning. Be flexible with the timing, length, and ingredients within your routine. Play with it until it feels satisfying to you and it is something you look forward to. No matter how busy you are, shift your priorities until you can find at least twenty minutes to yourself daily. After you've played with this for a while, if it still isn't working for you feel free to let it go. Remember, we are never forcing anything again! If something else strikes you as the perfect cornerstone shift, definitely implement that instead or in addition to the daily routine.

Chapter 9: Deep Play

Whenever we do anything, we either want to do it or we do not want to do it. This is the difference between want-power and willpower. Willpower comes from a place of obligation. You may want the result that the thing you are doing will bring you, but you do not want to be doing the thing itself. This is ends-justifies-the-means thinking. While in the midst of doing an action from pure willpower, you may feel resentment, exhaustion, depression, obligation, self-denigration, or more unpleasant emotions. Examples of doing something on willpower alone and the emotions that might follow are working a job you absolutely hate in order to earn money for a family (depression), doing your roommate's dishes when you've already asked him to please be more cleanly (resentment), or getting up in the middle of the night for the eleventh time with a newborn baby (anger). And let's not forget about dieting! Dieting is something we don't want to do (no one loves skipping wedding cake or ice cream at the beach), but we do it anyway because we want the end result. Dieting gives us feelings of exhaustion and self-disgust. The only way to deprive ourselves of the things we really want is to convince ourselves that we don't deserve them through the use of self-denigration. An ends-justifies-the-means approach to achieving a goal will bring with it emotional chaos. It will always diminish the end result. The result will bring with it very little satisfaction. Once the goal is achieved, another goal will take its place and the cycle will continue. Besides running out, willpower causes pain and suffering in the meantime. When operating from a state of willpower the mind is focused on the future. I have heard that the definition of hell is wanting to be somewhere else other than the present moment. So as much as possible we will try to operate on want-power which is available in the present moment.

Operating on want-power is the opposite of ends-justifies-the-means thinking. It is all about the journey, not the destination. Finding satisfaction in each present moment is the goal. Let's break down want-power into three categories: acceptance, satisfaction, and deep play.

At the low end of the spectrum is a type of want-power called *acceptance*. Acceptance occurs when the enjoyment level of an activity is quite low. For example, many people have jobs that they are not passionate about and everybody has to do things in their day that are menial and routine. But that doesn't mean these jobs or tasks have to be completely void of any joy. When washing the dishes one might enjoy the feeling of the warm water on her hands and take pride in being able to provide for herself and her family a clean-living environment. When filing papers in a back office one might enjoy the cool breeze of the AC on her cheeks, the peace and quiet of the empty room, and the warm smiles of coworkers as they come and go. While stuck in traffic one might enjoy a time to listen to a podcast with no other obligations. This is a state of acceptance, where the primary thing one is doing is not necessarily what she would have chosen to do if presented with other options, but she is able to do it with some amount of joy simply by bringing consciousness to that task.

A higher level of want-power is the state of *satisfaction*. Satisfaction occurs when the enjoyment level of a task is high. However, it is not enough for one to simply enjoy something to be satisfied by it. Many people enjoy getting drunk, binge-watching television, and overeating. But these activities lead to very little satisfaction. That is because they are generally performed without consciousness. Remember these are generally below consciousness activities. On the other hand, something like spending time with a toddler, which requires great attention to the present moment and can be quite enjoyable, will lead to true satisfaction for a caregiver. A career that one enjoys and brings her best to will require a great deal of consciousness and lead to high satisfaction.

The third state, and the highest level of want-power, is something we all wish we had more of. This is the state of deep play. In deep play the enjoyment level is highest of all. But again, it is not enough for just the enjoyment level to be high. When something has a very high enjoyment level but requires no consciousness, it could be addictive. Sugar, nicotine, and cocaine are examples of very enjoyable substances that, when used without consciousness, can lead to addiction. Deep Play, on the other hand, is a state of extreme consciousness combined with ecstatic joy. In this state, one is in a euphoric mood. Concentration is 100% in the here and now. The most creative and joyful aspects of the inner self are awakened. This is related to but slightly different from a flow state. One may be in a flow state with very little joy, such as when solving a problem to resolve an emergency situation. A person is in a flow state when the difficulty level of a task is very high but so is the skill level of the person doing the task. Deep play, however, requires the additional element of joy. When someone is in deep play, they are doing what they were called to this Earth to do.

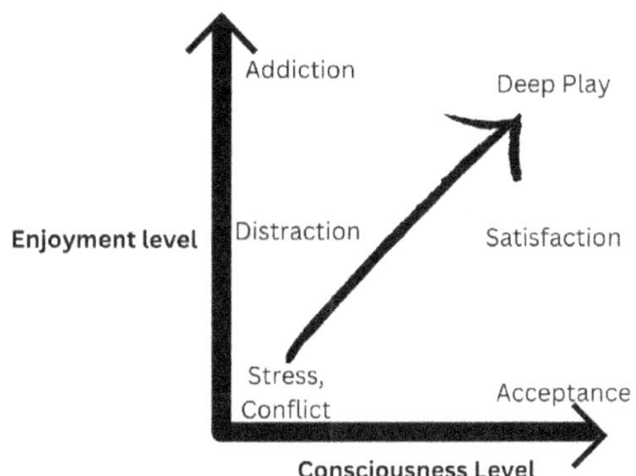

As you can see in the above diagram, when we are at a low level of consciousness and a low level of enjoyment there is much stress and conflict. (Such as working a boring job and wanting to be somewhere else.) If the enjoyment level increases but the consciousness level does not (by doing below consciousness behaviors), the tendency is toward addiction. (Such as unconscious eating or drinking). On the other hand if enjoyment is low but consciousness is very high, we can find acceptance in even the most unpleasant situations by turning our attention to the present moment. The best-case scenario is when consciousness and enjoyment are very high. This is deep play.

When we are in a state of deep play, we are able to do our best work in the world. This is where we are doing what we were put on this Earth to do. You will know when you are in deep play when time has no meaning, thoughts of the past or the future fall away, your emotional state is elevated, and the result of whatever you are currently engaged in will be to bring greater harmony, peace, and love into both your inner world and the outer world. This is when you are fulfilling your truest calling, your dharma.

Doing what lights you up and challenges you, with great consciousness, is the only way that you will bring to Earth the great thing that you were designed to bring. If you spend the majority of your day on things that do not feel like deep play you will never ever feel satisfied and you will always turn to something quick and easy to "fill you up." Whenever you find yourself in a situation to which you cannot bring acceptance you will start to crave an escape. You will look for something to bring a bit of enjoyment into an otherwise miserable situation. This is when Hunger strikes. That is why it is imperative that if you cannot make peace with the present moment, you change it. Sometimes we don't have a lot of choices, like getting stuck in traffic, or having to sit through hours of boring classes in order to be able to do the job we really want to do. In those cases we must strengthen our ability to bring acceptance into the present moment. Other times we absolutely must make a change.

Knowing when to make changes requires listening to biofeedback as we discussed in chapter eight. If your whole body is screaming "YES" and yet you continue to sit on the sidelines you are going to have a very hard time finding acceptance in the present moment and you definitely won't experience deep play. Likewise, if you find yourself day after day going to a job that drains your soul, you will struggle to find acceptance and it will be nearly impossible to ever find deep play. The best way to keep the cravings to drop below consciousness alive is to be at war with the present moment. And that is why diets will always fail. Diets are internal wars between an ironclad will and endless hunger. And I don't care how intuitive you are, your intuition is always going to tell you to eat more in order to escape the suffering that occurs from being in a situation which you cannot accept.

Again, I want to emphasize that the journey of a thousand miles starts with one step. You do not need to rush out and quit your job or anything else that you don't enjoy doing. Instead, drop small things that your body responds "no" to and add small things that your body says "yes" to. Additionally, bring more consciousness to the things in your life that you enjoy very little. By doing so see if you can start to enjoy the present moment even in challenging situations.

One student of mine liked her job for the most part but hated the hours per day she had to spend on emails. She felt like she never had enough time. After learning these principles she decided to only respond to emails for a set amount of time. She could bring acceptance for one hour, as long as she knew there was an end in sight, and she would still have enough time to complete the other tasks she needed to get done before closing time. Since she was no longer burnt out from responding to emails, she started to find her sales numbers were improving as she was able to really have fun while attending to her clients. But it didn't take long before the people sending emails were making second and third requests and CCing her manager. Soon her manager had a conversation with her. But instead of being upset, the manager said she had seen a spike in the employee's performance recently while also noting many emails left unattended too. She suggested maybe getting some extra help to relieve the employee of some of her clerical work so she could focus on the tasks where she really shined. In this case she did not need to make any major changes. A few small tweaks and a willingness to say no were all that it took.

I saw the principle of only making small changes in order to eventually have the big ones made for you illustrated in my husband a few years back. He was out of work, and I was pregnant. I repeatedly urged him to look for work. He took a job he wasn't sure he would like at my insistence that something was better than nothing. He is an independent contractor and accustomed to being able to set his own schedule. As a diehard surfer, a flexible schedule was a non-negotiable for him, since surfing can only be done when the conditions all line up. Even though it would have worked out fine for him to do his work with a flexible schedule on this job, the contractor didn't allow it. The contractor demanded that all subcontractors start at the same time. One morning I saw my husband packing his lunch and realized he was going to be late. "You need to leave now!" I pushed him. He said that having a nutritious lunch was more important than being on time. A few days later the surf was good, and he decided to stay home for the morning and complete his work later in the day even though the contractor said he needed to be there in the morning. Once again, I was upset with him. This happened a couple more times before he was told his services were no longer necessary. As you can imagine, I was more than a little upset at that point! He assured me that the right job was out there for him, and he didn't need to compromise his values to find it. Within two weeks he had another job. It paid better, offered as many hours as he wanted to work, had a completely flexible schedule, and included amazing perks. In this case he didn't need to quit his job, but it was taken away from him when he refused to say "yes" when his body was screaming "no." When this happens it is always because the universe has something even better for us. My husband, who is much better at trusting and staying true to himself than I am, had no problem believing that all he had to do was honor his desires and the rest would fall into place. He ended up having the highest earning year of his life in the year that followed.

Homework 6:
Answer the following questions in a journal (or a voice note):
- Where do I experience deep play?
- Where do I find myself wanting to be in a different place or time?
- Can I find acceptance in those moments?
- If not, what changes need to happen in order to at least find acceptance even if I can't get to satisfaction?
- Where am I dropping below consciousness in order to find temporary enjoyment as an escape from suffering?
- How can I create more moments of deep play?
- Where do I see addictions/attachments in my life? Can I bring more consciousness to those things?

Part II - Making Internal Changes

Life is filled with unpredictability. Like it or not, we cannot control every variable. Every day each one of us will face situations that we would rather not face. Whenever this happens, the only choice we have is a choice in how we respond. Most of the time we have an emotional reaction based on conditional subconscious programming. As soon as something bad (or good) happens, we already have attached a story to it. Let me illustrate this with a couple of examples.

I have a friend who deals with anxiety. Whenever her husband goes on a business trip she worries he might be cheating on her. Even though my friend logically knows her husband is faithful and he has given her no reason to mistrust him, she becomes very agitated and demands constant texts and check-ins from her husband. There is a story playing in her head about what might be going on. This is obviously very uncomfortable for her and not at all appreciated by the husband. In this case her suffering is not caused by her husband's actions but rather the story she is telling herself about her husband's actions.

Sometimes a situation inherently has much pain attached to it, but we often make it worse by attaching a story to it. For example, if I lose someone close to me, I will certainly experience great grief. But thoughts like, "I'll never be able to go on without her. My life is ruined. I will probably be the next one to die. This means I can never be happy again," will cause additional suffering.

There are two kinds of suffering we are talking about here. Suffering from painful things (say, the death of a loved one) and suffering from the story we tell ourselves about things. In Part I of this book we covered the topic of making changes to avoid having so many painful stimuli in our lives. And in Part III we will discuss how to deal with the painful things that are unavoidable. But this chapter is all about putting an end to the suffering that is caused by our thoughts. So the tools I'm going to share with you are extremely useful when we start to fall into the second kind of suffering, suffering caused by the stories we tell ourselves. When we can keep our thoughts from causing unnecessary pain, we can eliminate much of the suffering that we generally would have used food or another below-consciousness behavior to try to forget .

64

Chapter 10: The STOP and FLIP Formula

The first step in eliminating unnecessary mental suffering is to become aware. We need to be aware that we are having thoughts or creating stories. Have you ever noticed yourself talking out loud? Everyone does this occasionally. But we are constantly talking to ourselves in our heads and most of the time have no idea this is happening. Noticing this mental conversation comes with practice. It is like a muscle; it takes time to train it. The more we practice mindfulness meditation the easier this will become. Remember the goal of any meditative practice is not to eliminate thoughts but to be aware that we are having them and then to have the choice on what to do with them. Just because the mind is thinking, "I can never be happy again," doesn't mean it is true. When we become aware that the mind is having this thought then we have the ability to change it.

Mindfulness meditation is so simple that it often gets overlooked. For our purposes the kind of mindfulness that we will investigate is awareness of thoughts. It is useful to practice this when you are not feeling emotionally overwhelmed. Sit or lay down in a quiet place and focus on your breathing. Think of your breathing like a clear blue sky. Think of thoughts like clouds in that sky. Notice as each cloud comes into your awareness and watch as it goes out. That is to say, simply become aware of the contents of your thoughts. Do not investigate them, do not try to solve any problems, do not get caught up in them. So your mindfulness meditation might look a little like this: "I'm breathing, I'm breathing. I have to send that email tonight. Oh I'm thinking about email. I'm breathing. I'm breathing. What will I make for dinner? Oh I'm thinking about dinner." Remember, the point is to catch yourself having thoughts, not to eliminate them. The reason this practice is valuable is that you will train your consciousness to be aware of thoughts so that when powerful emotions strike, you will not have to be drawn into the story in which your mind spins around those emotions.

Whenever a powerful emotion is coming on it is imperative to pause and give your consciousness a chance to recognize what the mind might be thinking. When you become aware that you are making up stories, a simple word makes all the difference. Simply tell yourself, "STOP!" You can even say it aloud. So as soon as you notice the emotions starting up, tune into your thinking and if you notice an unhelpful story, tell it to STOP. We tend to have the same tapes that play the same tracks over and over, just with different spins. If you find yourself having a conversation with someone in your head STOP. If you notice yourself criticizing someone or dwelling on how you were wronged STOP.

The brain does not do well with an open circuit. Have you ever forgotten the name of something, and it drove you nuts until days later, seemingly out of nowhere, the name pops into your head when you were not even thinking about it? This is partly because the brain never let the thought go. It kept that track open on play in the subconscious until it could be completed. Likewise if you interrupt your thoughts midstream, the brain is going to fight to go back. Especially if you STOP your thoughts mid-sentence, the brain gets super agitated at this! So giving yourself something else on which to place your attention is very helpful. For this a grounding meditation is powerful.

This grounding meditation is super simple and can be done quickly from anywhere. Simply notice things around you, sights, sounds, textures, taste and smells. For example: "My Mother is such a… STOP… my shoulders are sore. The wind is blowing loudly right now. There is a photo of a fish on the wall. My coworker is wearing a lovely pink shirt." Then go on to the next step: flipping the story.

This is my favorite part of the process. Once you've been able to stop the story and capture your emotional state, then you are able to create the opposite of the emotion inside of you. Emotions create polarity. They will always seek their opposite to neutralize them. This is why when we feel down, we want to do something like eating a cookie to bring ourselves back up. So finding a way to create an opposite emotion within ourselves is super important. This is where flipping the story comes in handy. The story that created the emotional suffering in the first place always has

Internal Negative Story	Flip the Script to Positive
I will never be happy again since my sister's death.	My sister wants me to have a happy life.
My boyfriend is too lazy to plan a date.	I want to spend quality time with my boyfriend because he is such an amazing person.
My husband is probably cheating on me right now.	My husband is in love with me and would never hurt me.
We can't afford the things we need to be happy.	The universe is faithful; it has always provided before and will continue to do so.

a flip side. Find the flip side and make it into a one or two sentence mantra. Here are some examples:

The brain is most certainly going to get pulled back into its thinking and storytelling. The idea of flipping the story is that you find something, rooted in fact rather than emotions, for the brain to attach onto. Then repeat this new, more useful thought as often as needed to retrain your subconscious programming. These flips become the go-to thoughts whenever the story starts back up. The entire process can be shortened into a simple formula.

1. Become conscious of the thoughts.
2. STOP the thoughts by grounding.
3. Flip the thoughts.

There is one more step in this process that will be necessary when you feel an emotion may overwhelm you. You may have to add this step to provide a quick exit route for the emotion. Breath.

Chapter 11: Breath

After you've completed the above steps, it may be necessary to allow the emotion to exit your body in a way that is safe and can be done anywhere. Breathing is the fastest path between the body and the mind. There are many things we do involuntarily (digestion, circulations, etc.) and many things we do by choice (talking, walking, etc.). But breathing is the one thing that is both autonomic and somatic (voluntary and involuntary). Which means it has the superpower of being a conscious action that has the ability to regulate involuntary actions, such as emotional responses. And it has the added benefits of being simple, quick, powerful, always available, socially acceptable everywhere, and free. To take advantage of this powerful tool I will suggest one super easy breathing technique.

Take a deep breath in through either the mouth or nose.
Fill up the belly with the breath, making it expand.
Slowly release the exhale through the nose if possible.
Try to make the exhale take twice as long as the inhale.
As you exhale, relax your jaw, shoulders and glutes.
Repeat.

Try it now. Inhale into the belly. Long slow exhale. Relax. Again. Long slow inhale, longer slower exhale. Relax. Even one breath will make a difference. You can repeat up to ten times or more if you want.

Now you are in a state where you can deal with anything that needs to be addressed or changed without the pull of strong emotions causing additional suffering. Don't be surprised if this takes some practice to get the hang of.

Let me illustrate how this process can be life changing with a story from a client. Lorie had been married previously before she met Mark. She fell in love with Mark but not his cigarette addiction. When she told him it was a deal breaker, he immediately quit. Their relationship was like a fairytale and within a few years Lorie was pregnant. But shortly after the baby was born, Mark went back to smoking regularly. Being sleep deprived and overwhelmed trying to work from home with a new baby, Lorie took it out on Mark a lot. She often reminded him that smoking was not going to work for her and she would not be able to tolerate it for the rest of her life. Shortly after the arrival of the baby, Mark seemed very uninterested in the relationship. He spent long hours at work followed by more hours with his friends. Even their friends and family on both sides were taking notice of how little Mark put into the relationship. Lorie asked Mark several times to please spend more time at home helping her with the childcare. They even went to counseling to discuss the issue. But still Mark maintained his distance. Lorie started a story in her head, a seemingly logical one, that went like this, "Mark is a very selfish person. He doesn't care about me and our child. He doesn't love us. He doesn't even like us." She began planning a way to leave him.

After learning these principles she started to notice that she had a choice. Since he refused to change his actions, she could either leave him in order to avoid the anger she felt toward him (remove herself from a triggering situation) or change her reaction toward his actions (not become triggered). She didn't want to split her family up, so she decided to work on her reaction toward him. This wasn't easy, but she started by bringing consciousness to her thoughts. She began catching herself in the middle of her thoughts about what a jerk her partner was. She interrupted those thoughts and asked if they were true thoughts. She quickly became baffled because when she met her partner, he was not a jerk at all. He was actually giving and generous. And she often observed him being generous with his time to others. So why would he be acting selfish toward her? She stopped the story and replaced it with something she knew to be true, even though it didn't ring true to her at the moment. "Mark is a generous and loving person."

After a time, when her emotions were calm, she approached Mark with a question. "I know that you are a generous and loving person. That is why I fell in love with you in the first place. But I also notice you have stopped being generous with your time toward me. Since I love you unconditionally, I will respect your decision not to spent time at home, because I know you must have a good reason for it. Would you be able to tell me your good reason for not being around as much as I need?" Upon hearing this Mark opened up a great deal. He expressed that he was certain she didn't love him anymore. He thought with his return to smoking that it was only a matter of time before she left him, just like she had left the previous husband and just like she had threatened. He didn't want to invest himself into a relationship that was doomed. He didn't want to get close to his child only to have the child torn away from him. So he had shut down his feelings toward her in order to protect himself. Lorie was able to see how she had contributed to the problem. Certainly Mark had his own healing work that needed to be done. But Lorie, by noticing and challenging the story she attached to Mark's actions, was able to bring about the change she needed and deserved. It took time, open communication, and a lot of consciousness on both their parts, but within days Mark was home in the evenings and on weekends again, helping more and more and within months not only was Mark contributing as much as Lorie wanted, he had also significantly reduced his smoking without her asking.

I love this example because it illustrates that even when the mental chatter in our head seems completely logical and believable it is rarely objective or true. So let's put these tools into action now.

Homework 7:
1. Practice STOPping unhelpful mental stories with the process described above:
Notice the thoughts.

STOP the thoughts.
Ground by noticing the here and now.
Flip the thoughts.

2. Practicing the calming breath

Part III Pain Management

One day when I was about five or six, I was helping my grandmother at the candy store she owned. After a couple of hours of work, she asked if I wanted a piece of candy. I told her no. I said I felt a little sick in my stomach. It then occurred to her that it was past my regular lunchtime, and I hadn't had anything to eat in a few hours. "Oh, Melanie," she said, "You're hungry! You have to realize that the feeling in your stomach is hunger, and you need to let me know that you need to eat when you feel that." I never realized until I had my own child that children don't know what they are feeling until you give it a name and a solution. Toddlers have to be trained to notice the need to use the bathroom. They can swim in cold water until they are shaking and have blue lips without realizing their need for warmth. They will cry and get fussy because they don't feel good but refuse to get out of the water, having no idea their upset is stemming directly from being in the water. One day I took my two-year-old to run an errand early in the morning before breakfast. It took longer than I planned. I was confused when he started getting really moody. I wondered if maybe he was getting sick. When I got home and saw the time, I knew instantly what the problem was even though he didn't. A few minutes and a peanut butter covered banana later and my son was happily entertaining himself.

Somewhere in early childhood we were taught what hunger feels like. We became really good at catching it early, before it got out of hand. We learned what the solution was and became proficient in feeding ourselves. We were taught to do this all with our basic and obvious needs. Unfortunately, no one taught us how to do the same with our other feelings, like emotions.

Do you consider yourself an emotional eater? The vast majority of people who eat more than their bodies physically need are eating in order to make some kind of feeling go away. But most of these people have no idea that they are even doing it. They just know they are uncomfortable, and food seems to fix the problem, at least temporarily. So all sorts of unpleasant feelings get labeled as "hunger." Just like a child must be taught to recognize physical sensations and translate them into actions, adults must learn to recognize our emotions and nourish ourselves in appropriate ways. Until we learn this skill, emotions will feel a whole lot like hunger, since that is one sensation we are very dialed into. In the same way that a child must recognize a body sensation, name that sensation as "hunger" and then appease their appetite, the processes of recognizing, naming, and appeasement of emotions is an essential skill set that must be learned if one is ever going to heal their relationships with food. In Part III we take a deep dive into the colorful world of emotions.

Emotions will arise in life. Not all of them will be pleasant. Life is hard. It is full of painful twists and turns, and it never turns out 100% happily ever after. In Part I we discussed how we can take control of our lives to minimize pain. Part II covered the idea of avoiding secondary suffering that our thoughts add to both benign and painful situations. Part III is about the harsh reality of being human. It will provide tools for handling the painful emotions that are inevitable in life.

Chapter 12: Acceptance

Emotions have gotten a bad reputation for far too long. Men aren't allowed to have them at all, and women are written off as "being hormonal" for having them. Like PDA, public displays of emotions are equally frowned upon at work or in public places. But spend any time with a child under the age of five and you will see frequent, often violent and loud, displays of emotions. Why? Because children haven't had emotions conditioned out of them like us well behaved adults have. Now, I'm not suggesting we throw ourselves on the floor and wail when we don't get the promotion we wanted. But what I want to convey is that emotions are natural. Moreover, emotions are helpful; they arise for a reason.

On the first day with a new therapist I left her office with a handout tucked into my purse. On the sheet of paper were all kinds of faces wearing all kinds of expressions and under each face was an emotion. *Happy, angry, embarrassed, anxious, etc.* I thought this was very silly. Surely, any adult human already knows what these words mean. But on my next visit when my therapist asked me, "So when x happened, how did that make you feel?"
I responded with, "Like I wanted to…" She stopped me. "No but try using a word from the list." I was shocked that although I knew exactly how I wanted to *respond to x*, I had no idea how I *felt* about x. That is because emotional intelligence is a skill. I recently saw a mom pick up her crying toddler after a benign fall from her bike. "How did that make you feel?" she asked. "Were you scared or embarrassed?" Wow! That little girl has an excellent head start on something many parents do not know must be taught to children.

Often, we are in a situation where it is not socially acceptable, or even safe, to express our emotions. For example, in an emergency situation the emotions of fear and panic are not useful. However, if one does not take time after the emergency has been resolved to process back through those emotions they will start to suffer from PTSD. I can remember a situation when I was on my surfboard in the ocean and a terrible rip current was sucking me quickly out to sea. I wasn't sure if I had the strength to get back in. I remember thinking, "Stay calm, breathe, you can panic when you hit the beach." I used all my training and made it safely to shore. As soon as my feet hit the sand, I flung my surfboard dramatically and collapsed to the beach crying. I'm sure it was quite a sight for the tourists walking by! But as I allowed the emotions to drain from my body a strange euphoria overtook me. I remember staying up late that night and dancing around a bonfire. All emotions are on one side or the other of a pole. To the point that you allow yourself to experience any emotion, it's equal and opposite emotion will find you in order to reestablish balance. That is why love always comes with heartbreak and loss is always the beginning of fullness.

Emotions are energy. Each emotion carries a vibrational frequency. Quantum physics is just catching up to this fact that has long been known in eastern traditions. Emotions are electrical signals running through the nervous system. What is electricity? Energy with a specific frequency. So whether you are a "sciencey" person or more on the woo-woo side, the fact is, each emotion has an energetic signature. When our mind is lost in the past or the future, there will normally be a low vibrational energy with it. The emotions of the past start with nostalgia and drop lower and lower into sadness, regret, guilt, shame and depression. The emotions of the future start with wanting, and move into worry, stress, anxiety and fear. The farther towards the end of the spectrum, the lower the vibration. When the mind is rooted in the present moment, the emotions have an upward trajectory starting with contentment and moving up to euphoria, joy, rapture, and love. All emotions are useful for providing information. Some emotions are more comfortable than others, but they are not more or less useful. We need to be careful to remember that emotions are energetic responses to stimuli. They are responses. Emotions are not goals or things to be avoided. They are the reaction to a stimulus. And a useful one at that.

We have been conditioned to believe that it is not just the display of emotions that is unacceptable ("Quit your crying or I'll give you something to cry about!") but that even the emotion itself is to be avoided. Hopefully with this new inclusive view on emotions you can start to see the benefits to having emotions. They are just information. And information is power.

Now it is time to start paying attention to our emotions. If you've been around the spiritual community for some time, you may have heard the idea of sitting with one's emotions. Unfortunately jargon like this can lead to a lot of spiritual bypassing. These words are often thrown around but end up bouncing off the intended recipient and falling away without much meaning at all. How does one "sit with" an emotion, exactly? And more importantly, why would one want to do this at all?

Sitting with emotions means allowing the expression of the emotions to take form within the body and to allow that form to be expressed through the medium of the body. Let me show you what that looks like in a really concrete way. For this we will use a powerful tool I call *body mapping*. Let's try it now.

Imagine a person, place, object or situation that you would react to with great joy. A beautiful sunset, a passionate kiss, your child's face. Describe it to yourself in great detail. Think through the whole situation, colors, location, the clothes you're wearing. Don't miss a thing. Now hold that feeling of joy in your body. Ask yourself the following questions:

-What muscles are tense right now? (Cheeks from smiling?)
-What muscles are relaxed? (Shoulders, belly?)
-Where is joy located in my body? (Face, heart area, gut, tips of fingers?)

- If joy was moving what kind of movement would it make? (Pulsing, swirling, expanding, compressing?)
- If joy had a color, what color would it be?

- If joy made a sound, what sound would it be making?

Okay, now take a snapshot. Perhaps for you, joy is a purple tingling in the tips of your fingers with the sound of trumpets playing. Wonderful! This is what I call your "body map" for joy. Chances are joy is going to show up for you again and again in a very similar way. This is joy's energetic signature, written across your body. This is why we have so many expressions like, "my heart leapt" or "my stomach dropped" because emotions inhabit our bodies in a very physical manner. After all, they are called "feelings" because we are feeling something in our bodies.

Body maps are fantastic ways to experience emotions because it makes them completely neutral. When Joy is just a purple trumpet playing in your fingertips, it isn't something you need to drink a bottle of wine to go looking for. You can revisit this sensation anywhere, anytime. And when sadness is just a green swirl in your low back with the sound of rain falling, you don't have to be overwhelmed by it or afraid of it. It is just a sensation. It will not overwhelm you. It will not devour you. You do not need to distract yourself with food. It is just energy moving through your body.

Once an emotional signature has a map, it will also come with directions on how you can move it out of the body. As we know from physics, energy cannot be created nor destroyed, only transformed. For example the energy of the wind is captured by wind turbines and stored as electrical energy in power banks. When the energy is needed, it can be drawn out and transformed into light energy to light a house. The same can be said for emotional energy. It can either be stored (like in a battery) or it can be used to do something. When emotional energy is stored, it goes into our physical tissues. That map you just made lives there, in your gut or your shoulders or your fingertips. And it will stay there, trying to work its way out, through a stomachache, shoulder pain, or neuropathy, unless you find another way to let it out. When people are under stress, their fight-or-flight system is activated. Adrenaline fills their muscles, and they are able to run more quickly and perform acts of superhuman strength. This is a great example of an emotion going into the physical tissues. Likewise, it is known that anger and blood pressure are related as well as grief and heart attack. So when an emotion fills the body, it will first fill our tissues much like a wind turbine sends the energy of the wind into a power bank. The last thing we want is for that energy to sit there unused. That energy will always find a way out, eventually. The body is not meant to be a long-term storehouse of energy but rather a conduit to do something with that energy. So when energy is not expressed immediately it will find a way to express itself eventually as dis-ease.

The really amazing thing about body maps is that when you follow the sensation deeply enough, it will also come with an expression request. Sometimes it is very quick. For example, the energy from being startled when a mouse runs by your foot will quickly exit the body if you let out a good yelp. That is emotional energy being converted into vocal energy. When you hear a good joke and respond with laughter, again that is emotional energy being transformed into movement and vocalization. Crying when sad and dancing at a joyful event are more examples of emotional energy transfer. The more quickly we can learn to express the emotion with either movement or sound the more quickly the feeling will exit the body. Sitting at a wedding reception table, too afraid to dance, while your heart is bursting with joy over the marriage of your friend, is a great way to create an energy blockage. And what will you do with the discomfort from an energy blockage? Go back to the bar or the dessert table. Likewise, stifling tears because you don't want to seem weak will eventually cause problems. And when those problems start to show their heads, food will seem like a good escape.

So let's go back to the map we made earlier for joy. Bring that feeling back up in your body. Picture your happy place; go back to feeling the sensations that arise in your body. Feel them deeply and bring even more descriptive words to these sensations. When you feel you've completely described this emotional signature, notice if your body wants to move. Do you want to sway, bop your head, or "jump for joy"? (Notice the language we use!) Also notice if any sounds want to be made: shouting, laughing, singing, etc. For some people it's as easy as a big smile and other more expressive people will want to have a living room dance party. There is no right or wrong. It might feel a bit weird. After all, these are very primitive neurological systems that are being triggered. It is the reptilian part of the brain that regulates our flight/flight or rest/digest response so you may feel yourself acting a bit animalistic. As mentioned before, sometimes it isn't the appropriate time and place to express our emotional energy. That is fine. Just wait until you are in a safe place and let it rip!

Most of the time we do a pretty good job at expressing our pleasant emotions, at least partially. But the unpleasant ones often get stored for later, either because it is not a socially acceptable or safe time to express them, or we are afraid to let them have their expression because the pain is too great. But those times are when it is most critical that we *do* allow the emotional energy to be converted into physical or vocal energy. Not doing so means that pain is being stored in our tissues and will eventually cause physical discomfort and disease. This is why yoga is often used for PTSD therapy. When the body starts moving, powerful emotions do too. Any type of physical exercise is effective for awakening and releasing stored emotions, but yoga is especially helpful because the movements are slow enough to allow the practitioner to notice the emotions coming back up and the setting is generally socially acceptable to cry or otherwise express emotional energy. Massage therapy and a type of rapid eye movement therapy called EMDR are also quite effective means of releasing stored emotions.

Another powerful tool all of us use from time to time to transform emotions into movement is food. Food is a part of every celebration and every wake. The reaching, the opening, the smelling, the stabbing, the chewing, the crunching, the slurping, the licking, the digesting—it is all energy transfer. For unpleasant emotions, food has a particularly useful bonus in that it is extremely pleasurable and allows us to forget about the emotion before it is done expressing itself. And now you see the problem. These not quite fully digested emotions are stored, causing disease or weight gain, which causes more emotions, which causes more eating, which causes more disease or weight gain. That jiggly part of your body that you dislike so much is literally a reservoir of unprocessed emotions that were too painful to feel so your body graciously agreed to store them away in your fat tissues. Your fat is your body's pain storage.

It is imperative, if we are ever going to end emotional eating, that we learn to feel our emotions and express them fully, as quickly as possible, in the way the emotions are requesting to be expressed. Here are some ways to express unpleasant emotions: crying, journaling, exercising, shaking, dancing, yelling, hitting, moaning, deep breathing, kicking, biting, swaying, EFT or Tapping, making art, playing an instrument, etc. Talk therapy is useful as well, but only when you are allowed to express your thoughts with great "displays of emotions" (again notice our language) such as yelling, cursing, raising a fist, etc. (Talk therapy is useful for working out solutions to problems and many other things, but those are different matters than transferring emotional energy.)

Homework 8:

Take the time to map an unpleasant emotion. Think of a time recently when you felt sad or disappointed. (For now, please don't go to the worst trauma in your life. We will talk more about that later. With big traumas sometimes the energy transfer can be so big that it is safest to work through big traumas with a trained professional or at least a trusted friend.) Once you've pictured the sad or disappointing event, then create a map exactly as we did previously by answering the following questions:

- What muscles are tense right now?
- What muscles are relaxed?
- Where is this feeling located in my body?
- If this feeling were moving what kind of movement would it make?
- If this feeling had a color, what color would it be?

- If this feeling made a sound, what sound would it make?

First realize this is just a sensation. A sensation is neither bad nor good. Be aware if you are adding any stories to the sensation. Continually bring your awareness back to the sensation and out of the story about who wronged you or the meaning of the negative event. Then ask yourself how your body wants to respond to the sensation it is experiencing. What type of movement or vocalization would feel best right now? And then do it! It might feel a bit weird at first, screaming into a pillow or shadow boxing in your bedroom, but trust it. The better you get at listening the quicker you can diffuse the emotion. And you'll start to get so good that you can do it without anyone noticing: running a sprint while on the treadmill, scrubbing the dishes extra hard, even scrunching and wiggling your toes fiercely under the table.

Once you've completed a body map and expressed the energy, just be still and notice how you're feeling. Then try a couple more emotions if you are feeling up to it.

Chapter 13: Reverse Body Mapping.

As mentioned before, emotional intelligence is a learned skill. Just like a child needs to be taught to listen and respond to body sensations such as when to pee, when to rest, and when to eat, we need to learn to listen to more subtle sensations telling us that we are having an emotional response.

When I worked as a bodyworker, I commonly saw people who thought they were completely relaxed and yet had no idea they were clenching their glutes or shoulders. When I would touch that area and ask them to intentionally try to relax where my hands were touching, they would be shocked and express that they had no idea they were gripping. And this happens on a more subtle level all the time. We don't notice the heat creeping up the backs of our necks, the clenching in our jaws, the butterflies in our stomachs, or the pressure on our chests. We go about our days ignoring our bodies and then wonder why we feel so hungry all the time. The body is in distress and the only way it knows how to get some relief is by asking for something comforting, like food, by using a sensation that we are very tuned into, like hunger.

Luckily, the solution is simple: reverse body mapping. Reverse body mapping is listening to the sensations in your body, reading their signature and giving them a name. Let me give you a couple of examples.

A few months ago I was having some strange health symptoms. Because I have a high genetic risk for ovarian cancer, I decided to google the symptoms of that type of cancer. I saw a list of twelve symptoms and realized I had every one of them. I made an appointment with my doctor for the following week and tried to put the matter out of my mind as there was nothing else that needed to be done at that time. The next day I was pushing my son on a swing when my mind started running wild with what-if's. Suddenly I had a moment of consciousness. I noticed my thoughts were making up a very big story. I started scanning my body to see the map. I noticed tingling in my arms and legs. I noticed pressure over my heart. I was seeing yellow. That is when I remembered that I had seen this emotional signature before when I was surfing in the biggest waves of my life. "Oh!" I thought excitedly. "This is adrenaline! I LOVE adrenaline!" Without much thought I instinctively started pushing my son higher on the swing, jumping and shouting between each push. He was delighted, and I was having a blast too. We giggled as I ran circles around the swing and dashed under him between pushes. Soon I was physically spent and the feeling, along with the scary story, were nowhere to be found. As I would later find out I did indeed have ovarian cancer but at that moment while pushing my son on the swing there was literally nothing that needed to be done and the fear was unhelpful at best and perhaps even worsening my condition.

Sometimes we don't know the exact name of the emotion even after we have read its signature. For example, I worked with a client who was frequently feeling the urge to get up and make trips to the breakroom for snacks throughout her workday. When I asked her to describe the feeling of wanting a snack, she said it was a cartoon character in the pit of her stomach saying, "Muhahahaha." She didn't know what to make of that, so I asked her to just call the sensation Jimbo. Whenever Jimbo showed up, she had a frame of reference for what was going on in her body. I asked her to see if Jimbo showed up at other times throughout the day, when she wasn't hungry. It turns out Jimbo was showing up all over. He showed up when she walked into her dark empty house after a long day at work. He showed up when she opened her inbox and saw an email she didn't want to deal with. He showed up when it came time to go to a party she promised to go to weeks before but no longer wanted to attend. The more she got to know Jimbo the more she was able to notice different shades of him. Sometimes he would also come with pounding in the heart, sometimes with bright flashing colors.

After a while, Jimbo started to look like different characters altogether. And the more nuanced they became the more she could identify them as separate emotions. There was loneliness, overwhelm, exhaustion, and more.

Reverse body mapping and forward body mapping work hand in hand. The more practice you have with forward body mapping the more familiarity you gain with the signatures of each emotion. Then when you are reverse body mapping, you can quickly read that signature and give it a name in order to identify what you are feeling. Reverse body maps are the key to ending emotional eating as we will soon see!

Chapter 14: Decoupling Hunger

Let's review our definitions of big "H" Hunger and little "h" hunger. When we are hungry (with a little h), the body genuinely needs food for its optimal physical functioning. When we are Hungry (with a big H) we need something for optimal mental, emotional, spiritual, or possibly physical function, but it isn't food. Because food can be a temporary solution to a big H hunger, we end up getting hunger and Hunger confused within our bodies. This is where body maps are hugely important: to decouple the sensation of needing food for physical function from needing something else for overall functioning. And although it does take a bit of practice, the process is simple.

When faced with a desire to eat the first step is to pause. For now we will call this sensation hunger, but that name might change. Map that sensation in your body. Create a detailed body map. Notice if this sensation still wants to be satiated through eating or if something else might be useful in moving the sensation through the body. If after a couple of minutes you still want to eat, eat. Eat exactly what sounds good. Eat mindfully, tasting each bite and enjoying the sight, sound, flavor, and texture of the food. Stop eating whenever you feel you've had enough. Now re-evaluate. Is the sensation still there? If so, eat some more. Once again, stop whenever you are ready. How is the sensation now? At this point if food has not taken away the sensation it is unlikely that this sensation was true hunger. No problem. Now you have a map of something that is not hunger. Just give it a human name like "Bob" for now and tuck it away. If the hunger went away after eating but returned quite quickly (in less than an hour or two), perhaps it was big H hunger after all, and you need something other than food to satiate yourself. Continue repeating this exercise each time you suspect you are hungry. You may recognize emotions right away or it may take you a while of using human names before you know what emotional name to call them. The more you practice with forward body maps the easier these reverse body maps will become because you will already know each emotional signature in your body.

I remember clearly the day the light bulb went on for me. I had been going to the kitchen five to ten times per day between the hours of 11 am and 4 pm for over two years. I could not understand why my body was sooo hungry. I was gaining weight. One day I decided to "sit with my Hunger." I made friends with it. I decided it wasn't a sensation to be satiated. I didn't need to erase it. Instead, it was a great teacher with information for me that I desperately wanted to learn. So I noticed where this Hunger was living in my body. It was in my chest. It felt like pressure from the inside out. I recognized it right away. This wasn't hunger, this was anxiety. I then "sat" with my anxiety. I traced its tentacles all throughout my body. I followed its movements; I felt its patterns. It was hard at first, very uncomfortable. But the more I practiced with it the more it lost its power over me. What used to be unbearable anxiety became nothing more than another sensation within my body. As I practiced mapping anxiety over and over it would start to have an expressive energy about it. It wanted to create! It wanted a worthwhile project; it wanted something to dump its energy into. That is when I first started writing. I haven't stopped. From that time, writing has been my most powerful anti-anxiety medication. I've noticed that sometimes writing isn't enough and I need exercise, fresh air, or simply to put my efforts into a different direction such as cleaning the house. Other times no action at all is required. Once I notice anxiety, I sometimes notice a story along with it. Sometimes I'm worried about money or relationships. In that case, once I become aware of the story it loses its power. I am able to use the techniques of Part II to STOP and Flip the story so the anxiety can drain from my body.

A fantastic exercise for mapping the signature of true hunger in the body is to simply delay eating once or twice. I absolutely do not suggest doing this on a regular basis. As mentioned, the urge to eat is important whether or not it is physical hunger. But as an exercise you can lean into that urge to eat for some extra time to find out what true hunger feels like. I suggest doing this when you're fairly certain you do need food, like when you haven't eaten for four hours or more, after an exercise session or at a regular mealtime when you haven't been snacking beforehand. Find a time when you are pretty sure you do need food and then wait an additional fifteen minutes, no longer than thirty minutes. Wait until you feel that sensation of emptiness in the belly. Make a really good map of this feeling and write it down to be sure you don't forget it. This is the signature of true hunger in the body. Whenever this signature shows itself, rest assured your body needs physical nourishment.

Homework 9:
1) Wait for a moment when you are truly hungry and map that sensation.
2) Map Hunger each time it strikes.
    a) If you're not sure what the sensation is, then give it a human name and be curious next time that sensation comes back.
    b) If you recognize the sensation as an emotional signature that you've already mapped, give it the name of that emotion.
    c) Whether you recognize the sensation or not, continue to map the emotion for as long as you can comfortably withstand. If you sense the need to move, vocalize or do something, follow that path!
    d) If the sensation does not dissipate after five to fifteen minutes and you still want to eat, eat! And definitely don't guilt trip yourself. Just keep practicing!

Chapter 15: Healing from Trauma

As we make progress along the trajectory of ending our craving to eat what no longer serves us, one of the sticking points for so many people is the memory of trauma. Whether one is clinically diagnosed with PTSD or not, the memory of trauma is one of the bigger challenges we will address. Since one definition of trauma is "something that overwhelms the central nervous system" it makes sense that when those memories are triggered in someone, they would turn to the first available means of comfort, often food.

When we talk about healing from trauma, we are actually talking about ending the emotional response that we continue to have in response to the memory of an event. The memory may be subconscious or conscious and the response may come with or without a physical response in addition to an emotional response. All humans experience some trauma. The amount of trauma is not important. The current imprint of that trauma is what we are interested in addressing.

Dr. Bessel van der Kolk, a leading PTSD researcher, says, "Trauma is not the story of something that happened back then. It's the current imprint of that pain, horror, and fear living inside the person now."

So the work of healing from trauma has everything to do with how we address the emotions associated with the memory of an event and not the event itself. The event is in the past. It cannot be changed. But the current imprint of that event can be healed. The good news is, we already know the methodology to do this work. Dr. van der Kolk teaches, "Trauma victims cannot recover until they become familiar with and befriend the sensations within their bodies. In order to change, people need to become aware of their sensations and the way their bodies interact with the world around them. Physical self-awareness is the first step." Or put another way, "Neuroscience research shows that the only way we can change the way we feel is by becoming aware of our inner experience and learning to befriend what is going on inside."

Lucky for us we have been working on this for a while now as we practice body mapping and reading emotional signatures. Now it is time to take this to the next level. The thing with big time trauma is that it goes above and beyond our normal everyday emotions and imprints itself deep within our tissues. Remember we talked about emotions as energies and how those energies go into our physical tissues and inspire us to make physical and vocal expressions. When we do not take these actions, those energies are stored away in physical tissues and stay there until expressed or the body forces them out as physical dis-ease and clinical disease. So our approach to addressing the emotional damage from trauma will involve the same ideas as addressing everyday emotions—feeling the energetic signature in the body and finding physical release. But because trauma goes very deep, we will need special excavation equipment. What follows is a toolbox filled with the tools useful for healing from trauma.

Because trauma can encode itself into the deepest parts of our physical being, it is not unheard of for people to have major medical responses such as seizures, heart attack, and more when doing this kind of healing. This is all just energy's way of pushing itself out. I have personally had deep bouts of weeping, migraine headaches, and nausea to the point of vomiting. You will need to listen to your physiological symptoms and know when to stop the exercise. Because of this reason it is always best to do this kind of work with a qualified trauma therapist. Check with your doctor before trying these therapies. Always follow the advice of your medical doctor. I have seen friends work together to support each other as they have worked through some of these therapies, but I cannot recommend trying these methods without a qualified practitioner. If in doubt, stop. You can revisit this work when you have the right help and when you are ready.

Here is the trauma healing toolbox.

1. Body Mapping.

> Of course we have already talked about this. Please refer to chapter thirteen if you need a refresher. In chapter thirteen I suggested not going to your darkest emotional places alone. I will suggest this again. Listen to your intuition about how much body mapping you can handle.

2. Bodywork.

> Bodywork such as massage, acupuncture, and reiki are excellent ways to move stored emotions out of the body. Try to find a therapist with trauma sensitivity training. The session can specifically focus on releasing trauma, or you might just get regular bodywork done to help keep energy moving. Remember to approach your session with a great emphasis on feeling what comes up. Stay present and treat the session as a meditation. Focus your attention on the physical sensation, both big and small. First focus on the big sensation, such as how good the strokes of the massage therapist feel on your shoulders. But then see if you can feel what is happening beneath the layers of skin, fat, muscle, blood, and bone. Can you become aware of the way energy is moving through your body? This is especially fun in acupuncture since a good acupuncturist will specifically place the needles to get energy flowing. See if you can feel its flow. Don't worry if at first you feel nothing at all. Just keep trying.

3. Yoga.

> Yoga is a fantastic way to combine attention to physical sensations with movement. The movement does not need to be fast. In fact, for working with trauma it may be better to go slow. This is because you want to have enough time to feel both the big and the small sensations. (For more study David Emerson has a fantastic book called *Overcoming Trauma Through Yoga: Reclaiming your body* .)

Again, I recommend finding a class with a trauma sensitive yoga instructor. You can also find trauma informed yoga classes on the internet. I suggest doing these at home videos with a trusted friend or qualified guide if you know your trauma is quite deep and until you are comfortable going there alone. Of course, consult your doctor before starting any exercise program.

4. EMDR: Eye Movement Desensitization and Reprocessing. EMDR is a way of combining talk therapy and movement, specifically eye movement, to process trauma. Rapid eye movement is thought to be a way of cataloging and filing away memories in a way that is useful to the body which does not allow those memories to continue to cause pain. EMDR capitalizes on the power of rapid eye movement by using it in conjunction with talking though traumatic memories. The results are powerful. There are tutorials for how to do this yourself on the internet but of course the best results normally come from working with a qualified therapist. And of course this is the safest way as well.

5. Neurofeedback. Neurofeedback is the use of brain activity monitoring devices (EEG sensors) to input that activity into a software program in order to provide real time feedback. Essentially, this is a big shortcut on body mapping which makes use of technology to give us instant feedback. Neurofeedback sessions are typically done in an office although it is possible to rent the equipment and do sessions at home. Just like learning any new skill you will need to practice. Neurofeedback is useful for those with PTSD because they can train themselves to shift from a hyper aroused state into a calmer one using the brain, not food or other drugs.

6. MDMA (methylenedioxymethamphetamine). There is a growing body of clinical research supporting the use of the psychedelic drug MDMA in

treatment of PTSD. I cannot recommend this therapy based on anything other than clinical research and anecdotal stories. As with any psychedelic medicine, one should be prepared by doing the work of the previous suggested therapies first. Then it is critically important that all psychedelic medication be done under the supervision of a qualified guide and in the proper setting. Please speak to a doctor before considering this option.

This is certainly not an exhaustive list of activities that will help open the body in order to detox emotional stores. Anything that involves energy transfer will work especially when the focus is to purge emotions. Some examples are, writing, chi gong, animal therapy, tantric sex, women's circles, and many more. When you find a modality and/or practitioner that you enjoy, stick with it until you no longer feel you can benefit from it. Whether you suffer from PTSD or not, it is a great idea to have a regular practice involving some type of intentional emotional energy transfer in order to regularly cleanse from the everyday minor traumas that everyone experiences.

Chapter 16: Body Image

Body acceptance is absolutely mission critical if we are ever going to end the battle with food and weight. As long as we keep fighting our bodies, we will fight a losing battle. Manhandling, coercing, and forcing are rarely the best ways to get anyone to do anything, so why do we do these things to our own bodies? If our bodies are ever going to stop crying for help (drop extra weight) they must first believe at a cellular level that their cries are being heard and lovingly addressed. The only way to do this is to accept that where our bodies are now is perfect, even if it isn't the ideal place for them to stay. We must be able to look upon our bodies with compassion and respect for all they provide for us.

I know what you are thinking, "You want me to accept my hypertension, type II diabetes, aching knees, and sore back? I'm just supposed to sit back and do nothing while I run my health into the ground?" I am not suggesting you "give up on yourself" nor "let yourself go." What I am suggesting is that you accept that your body is doing the best it can with what it is given. You are not broken at all. Your body is not screwed up. If your weight is causing you physical distress, it is your body's way of getting your attention. It is under-resourced and using primitive coping strategies to solve a problem. Think of the way a baby cries when it is hungry, uncomfortable, or needs attention. No loving mother has ever said, "My stupid baby, she just keeps crying. She must be defective; I can't stand to be around her. I wish I had gotten a different one." And yet we say similar things about our bodies all the time when in reality our bodies are only trying to send us signals that something is wrong, and they need our help.

Body image is a spiritual issue. We know in our heads that our worth has nothing to do with our looks. But we don't feel this in our hearts, so we continue to suffer.

Healing a poor body image is going to require healing our deepest held beliefs about who and what we are. This section is going to get a little deep. Just hang with me. Concrete activities are coming. So even if these spiritual concepts I'm about to discuss seem a little out of reach, just take what you can and come back for the rest when you are ready.

Here is a harsh reality. The perfect body does not exist. Even if you lose the weight, you won't be happy when you get there. There will be wrinkles, sunspots, stretch marks, sagging skin, unwanted hair, deflated breasts, the wrong kind of butt, lack of muscle, an imperfect nose, or whatever perceived imperfection may arise. Even if you spend the hundreds of thousands of dollars you need to undergo invasive and painful procedures to change these things, you're still going to want more. Better clothes, a better car, a more prestigious career, a more supportive partner, it is literally endless. This is because a poor body image points to something much deeper: a low self-worth. When our internal evaluation of ourselves is low, no amount of weight loss, plastic surgery, or money will help us. These things are external. We need an internal solution to an internal problem. The solution starts with a very counterintuitive shift in thinking: you are not better than anyone.

Here is the thing, a poor self-worth comes from measuring ourselves against others and falling short. But the underlying belief in comparison is the problem. We believe that if only we looked like her then we would be better. Better than what? Better than all the people who look like us now? Do you see how this comes from ego? It is a desire to look or be better than others. We believe there is a way for one human to be superior to another. Can you see that the root thinking is that same thinking that causes acts of racism, sexism, and war? They all come from low self-worth and a belief that some kind of person is better than another. In reality we are not comparing "apples to apples" as the saying goes. Does a pine tree compare itself to an oak and wish it had those long, beautiful branches? Maybe the oak is looking out at the pine wishing it had such fullness in its bows. Does the hammer wish it had the screwdriver's slender trunk and the screwdriver wish it had the power of the hammer? This is ludicrous. *Each human is unique for a reason.* We each have a very specific function to fulfill in the ever unfolding of the universe. We were designed as unique tools to fulfill that specific function. Each of our features, from our personality right down to our varicose veins, were given to us for a reason. Changing ourselves so that we are more like someone else actually weakens us and makes us less effective at achieving our mission on planet Earth. If you believe you are worth less than someone, then you also believe in a hierarchy that doesn't exist.

Now let's take it a step deeper. In reality, there is no one to be better than. Let's think back to all the meditations we've been doing so far in this book. We have been working so hard to separate our thoughts from our true selves. By this point you might be starting to understand that you are not your thoughts but rather the consciousness that bears witness to those thoughts. You are more than a body and a brain. You are the consciousness that animates them. You are spirit. I am spirit experiencing this physical realm as a phenomenon called Melanie. We are all spirit. That spirit experiences itself through billions of conscious beings. But in reality, we are all one.

Think of it like this. In the beginning there was nothing but pure consciousness (or God, spirit, whatever you want to call it). Having nothing but consciousness, there was no way for consciousness to know its nature. There was no contrast. Like a fish not knowing water is wet, consciousness needed some medium through which to experience itself outside of itself. So it split itself into black and white. I love the Biblical narrative of this. First consciousness split itself into light and dark. Then it split itself into all sorts of diversity. Finally consciousness split itself into beings capable of knowing that they are consciousness and yet experiencing the diversity of consciousness as separate from themselves. A human is a medium for consciousness to experience itself. Have you ever said, "I said to myself…." Who is the *I* and who is the *self*? *I* is the consciousness that is aware of the human self.

So if you're still with me (and don't worry if I lost you, come back whenever you feel the pull to this and try again), you can see how we are all just one single consciousness. There is literally no way for one human to be better than another human; we are all the same thing. And I don't mean we are all clones. I mean we are literally just different shadows of the same figure. We are the same photo with different filters. We are the same painting being viewed in many different lights. No one can be ugly unless I am ugly. Likewise, I can't be beautiful unless all are beautiful.

It is confusion then that causes poor self-worth and body image. It is an identification with form. It is the belief that *I* am this body and that this body is *me*. You are the steward of your body. You are to treat her with great care and compassion. You are here to protect and serve her. And she is here to be your vehicle by which you will have powerful human experiences. There is no right or wrong, good or bad, better or best.

When I got cancer, I felt great sorrow for my body. I did not feel sorry for *myself*. With each chemotherapy session I apologized to my body for putting her through it and thanked her for hanging in there yet again. When my body felt weak, I honored her requests for rest. When she wanted to exercise, I allowed her to try her best and gave her accolades for trying even when she had to bow out shortly after starting. When it was time for surgery, I was scared that the scar would be very disfiguring. I went onto an internet support group for my type of cancer and asked the women if they would be willing to post pictures of their surgical scars. I was overwhelmed at the number of women, many of them elderly and with lots of belly fat, who were willing to post photos of their midsections with scars running from the breastbone to the pubic bone. Not only were these women willing to post photos of their large bellies, but they were also proud of them. Because these women had been through hell, and like warriors, they had made it to the other side, scared but more alive than ever. They were proud of their strength as evidenced in their scarring and no amount of belly fat could take away that pride. These women loved their bodies for reasons having nothing to do with aesthetics.

The truth is that when I see my bald head, lack of eyebrows and eyelashes, bags under my eyes, sagging skin, and rounded shoulders I do not see a sexy young woman in the way our culture defines "sexy." But I still feel a sense of pride in my body for all that it has done and continues to do. I feel great compassion. I feel tenderness and love for my body. And even though pop culture "sexy" Melanie has disappeared, I still feel sexy in that I have a sex drive and a sex life. When I first lost my hair, it was a shock and I mourned the loss. But soon I found that people, including myself, could see my true strength more clearly without the hair. Many new mothers experience this same type of body compassion and pride after having undergone the experience of building a human inside their bodies. Once a woman knows what her amazing body is capable of it becomes harder and harder to hate the stretch marks that came along with such an accomplishment.

Healing the way we view our bodies and our worth in general takes three massive paradigm shifts. First, we must heal our beliefs about why we are here in the first place. Understanding that we are each unique because we have a unique purpose is the first step. Second is understanding that our individuality is only a different expression of our commonality. Therefore, if beauty exists in you, then it is only a mirror showing what exists within me. Lastly, we must understand that a body (as well as a mind, career, bank account, or anything else belonging to "me") is only something I get to steward, care for, nurture, and enjoy, but it is not *me.* Like a cat adopted from an animal shelter, I am charged with its care, and I often experience both pleasure and pain from living with it, but it is not who I am nor does it say anything about my intrinsic value. I will summarize these three belief shifts as follows:

1. I have a unique body on purpose to complete a unique purpose.

2. We are all the same one-consciousness experiencing itself through unique human experiences. No one has more value than another because we are all one.
3. I am not my body but the loving caretaker of it.

Agreeing with these statements is one thing, but to truly embody this new perspective we will need lots of practice. The following activities are concrete ways of working toward embodiment of these new ideas.

Chapter 17: Body Image Activities

Changing the way we view our bodies and our self-worth in general is going to take work. Like a bodybuilder, we must train often and consistently. The good news is that the training works! Lift the weights and you will see the muscles. In the same way, completing these activities will have a huge impact on your self-worth if you commit to doing the work. Here are eight powerful activities for rewiring toxic thinking around the concepts of body and self-esteem. I suggest trying one or two per week. Don't rush this process. If the activity feels really good, keep it up. If not, drop it. You can always try it again later. There is no particular order here so start with whatever sounds the most fun and resonates with you the most.

1. Break Up with the Scale

   This is the easiest and most fun activity. Find your scale, and find a hammer. Bust it up into little pieces before depositing it in the trash. Scales are 1000% done in your life for good! You can know your weight when you go to the doctor. Period.

2. Thank the Thighs

   For this activity you will need to be completely naked or in a bathing suit/underwear. Get comfortable, either in front of the mirror, on your bed, or in the bathtub. Find the area of your body that you dislike the most (belly, thighs, butt, etc.). Gently, with great love, touch that part of your body. Hold it, rub it, stoke it. Get out some massage oil or lotion and give that part of your body a loving massage.

   Think of all the times food was there for you, when you didn't have the strength to face the pain. Think of the times you ate away the pain. Thank that body part for holding all this pain so you didn't have to. Send pure love to that body part for all the protection it has given you. Apologize for the hatred and disgust you've directed toward it. Forgive yourself, you didn't know any better. Promise to treat it better, loving it, and no longer demanding it hold your emotions. Promise to be the steward of the body, mind, and emotions, to care for your wounded emotional self so this body part doesn't have to store all that pain anymore. Practice this activity as often as you want until you really do feel a strong appreciation for that part of your body. Revisit this activity any time you start feeling negative toward your body.

3.   The First Time in the Mirror

Stand in front of a full-length mirror either in your underwear or completely naked. Imagine you are from a different planet. You've never seen a naked body before. You have no idea of the words "belly" or "arms" or any other body part. Neither do you know what any other humans look like, so you have nothing to compare this body against. Begin to investigate your body with deep curiosity. Feel the soft parts, the ridges, the folds.

Describe them with words like "magical, sparkling, delicious, incredible, revolutionary, juicy, joyous, soft, supple, cuddly, distinguished, marked, noteworthy, interesting, defined, textured, etc."

When you are finished grab your favorite lotion or body oil and give yourself a loving massage. Continue describing and appreciating each body part.

4.   Turn Your Light On

Turning your light on refers to tuning into your most confident, flirtatious, and sexy self. This is important if you are in a partnership, dating, single, or not even looking. This is for YOU, not anyone else.

Choose a non-threatening event where you will be with friends, such as a house party, meeting friends for drinks, or even going to a church service. Pick out clothing that flatters your shape. If appropriate, show a little extra leg or shoulders, whatever parts you feel most confident showing. Buy a new outfit if you can afford it. Don't get it at the discount store. Get something of high quality that really looks and feels fashionable and flattering. Spend a little extra time on your makeup and hair. It doesn't have to be darker, just more to your liking.

Look yourself in the mirror before you leave and say, "I'm going all in!"

Now, the goal is to be your most authentic self. Who would you be if you already knew everyone adored you? How would you act if you were a famous celebrity that everyone was always trying to get close to? If you could say anything and everyone would hang on your words, what would you say? That is who you are tonight!

In order to get the confidence flowing, start by asking someone all sorts of things about themself. (Bonus points if you've never met this person.) People love to talk about themselves. Pay special attention to remembering any new names and call people by their names a few times. For a while don't talk about yourself at all. Get really curious about the people around you, as if they were the most interesting people you've ever met. Bring them out of their shells. This part is meant to bring confidence. It works best when it is not fake but rather when you take a genuine interest in people's unique stories. This is a SURE way to endear new people to you.

You will be feeling on fire within an hour. Keep at this part until you feel wonderful.

When you are ready, let down your guard a bit. Drop the instructions here and just be yourself. If there is music and you want to dance, DO IT. If the dishes are being cleaned up and you want dessert, ORDER IT! Crack jokes, give inappropriately long hugs… be 100% yourself. Follow your intuition boldly. Try to do this without the aid of alcohol, or at least keep alcohol to a minimum, so that you are drawing on true confidence.

AND… if there is someone there you're attracted to, even if it's your long-time partner, be as flirtatious as you naturally can be (if it's appropriate). The idea is to push yourself to express your authentic self outside of your comfort zone, not to mimic anybody else. So don't fake any flirtatious behavior or any other kind of behavior, just let your body do and say what it wants to without the constant censoring or wondering what people will think.

Note: Not everyone is going to like your most authentic self. This is how you know you are doing it right! The more you come into your uniqueness, the more people who are scared of showing up to their own authenticity will be jealous. You will make them really uncomfortable. This is fine. Some relationships may naturally fall away. Let them go. New relationships will replace them with people who, like you, are unafraid of acting according to their individuality. These are your people. Let the haters go.

5.   Social Media Curation

Go through your Instagram/Facebook/TikTok feeds and block every social media account that promotes diets, workouts, or just triggers you to feel bad about your body. Girls looking hot in bikinis? BLOCK! From here on out your social media is your go-to for inspiration, not triggers!

Instead start following some women whose bodies you might not have seen as beautiful before you really opened your eyes. Fill your feed with examples of people who you admire for reasons beyond their bodies. This is one of the most powerful shifts you can make if you are a heavy social media consumer. Keep this up until your social media feed is 100% filled with inspiration and never makes you feel bad or jealous. Don't forget to block and report ads for things like diets and workout programs promising to make you thin.

Here are a few suggestions to get you started:
@Jesselleking
@megancarole
@amandittaplus
#normalbody
#bodyacceptance
#instavsreality

6.   Affirmations on the Mirror

On your bathroom mirror take a whiteboard marker and write your favorite things about yourself. Leave just enough space to be able to do your hair and makeup. Do the same on your full-length mirror. Even better, cover the full-length mirror with a sheet and only use it when you really need to check your outfit. Better still, get rid of it all together. It really is possible to match your top to your bottom without a mirror. The idea is to stop looking at ourselves as much as possible. Mirrors that show every wrinkle, roll, and freckle have only been around for less than 200 years. Inspecting ourselves down to the last detail really isn't necessary and if you find yourself feeling bad about your body after doing it, let it go!

7.   Pat on the Back Journal

This is best done on a note in your phone or a notepad that is always nearby.
Each time you do something you feel good about, jot it down. It's that simple. If you want, you can even add how it made you feel.
Examples: Wrote a perfect email to my client, feeling bad ass!
Made time for my morning routine. Feeling centered.
Put together a cute outfit. Feeling unstoppable!
Try to write down ten pats on the back per day for a week. You will be amazed how easy this activity becomes after a few days. We have trained our brains to be hypercritical of ourselves. This activity trains us in the opposite kind of thinking. The truth is that all of these good things have been here all along, but we haven't been looking for them. Have you ever bought a new car only to see that same make and model everywhere? What is going on with that? Of course those cars have been there all along, but we were not looking for them before. That is what we must do with our own successes, train our awareness of them. Stick with this activity until you become consciously aware of all the little successes you achieve each day, even without writing them down.

8.   Notice Beautiful Women

This is about seeing your own beauty being reflected back to you. Imagine each woman you see is a mirror. If you feel badly about yourself, you are going to see the flaws in others. When you are feeling good, you will see their beauty. It's time to intentionally look for beauty.

Intentionally notice women. If you want, you can sit on a park bench and spend dedicated time on this activity or just work it into your normal day, at work, at the grocery store, etc.

Look for their beauty. Especially in women you might consider "overweight." Notice the way they move, the color of their skin, the way they've given attention and care to their hair and makeup.
Make this a regular practice. Especially if you notice your first thought is something negative about someone's body. A negative thought about a person's body is just a negative thought about yourself. Use the STOP procedure.
STOP the thoughts.
Ground yourself.
Feel what that thought feels like in your body.
Change the thought by looking for something beautiful in her.

I was recently at the beach sitting close enough to another couple that I could hear their conversation. Two young women with average sized bodies walked in front of us wearing very tiny bikinis. Because of the work I have done, my first thought was, "Wow, look at those beautiful butts!"
The man next to me commented to the woman he was with, "Looks like those women are looking for attention. And the woman replied, "That's just gross. Some people shouldn't be showing that much skin."
Their comments were very telling of what was going on in each of their subconscious minds. The man was uncomfortable with the fact that his eyes were drawn to the young women, thus his comment about them wanting attention. The woman obviously felt her own body was gross; she wore her swimsuit cover up even in the water.
Whatever we project onto others comes from some dark thing we are hiding inside ourselves. When you feel those judgmental thoughts coming up just notice them. Give

yourself grace. Then flip the story. This will take some practice but with time it will be one of your most powerful tools for healing repressed pain.

Remember, the point of the above eight practices is to help you to embody the ideas that
1. Our individuality is our strength
2. We are all one
3. We are not our bodies nor our minds

These are massive statements that can be easy to throw around without them meaning much at all. As you do the above activities be sure to return to your journal now and then to reflect on how your beliefs are shifting. Can you write the above statements in your own words? Can you give examples of how the statements ring true for you? Can you explain these concepts to a friend? When expressing truths about our deepest nature it is hard to use human language to explain them away without trivializing them. Just continue to come back to these concepts now and again as you feel your self-worth and body image shifting.

Part IV Caring for the Body

There is a very good reason I have saved this topic for the end of the book. We often look at weight as a physical problem. So we try to address it using physical solutions, like eating less or moving more. When in reality weight is almost always more than just physical. Once you have addressed the spiritual, mental, and emotional causes of extra weight, then you can begin to dive into the last remaining, and least important issues: what we eat and how we move. I want to stress that if you have not done the work in the first three parts of this book, then skipping ahead will prove unhelpful at best and possibly very frustrating. If you have not read the first three parts of this book and invested time and thought into the homework, I highly suggest going back and doing so before reading this part of the book.

Before jumping into a discussion about how, when, what, and how much to eat we need to review a very important topic: how to distinguish between physical needs and mental/spiritual/emotional needs that show up as physical urges.

Physical urges are needs, but not necessarily physical needs. A physical urge, such as the urge to eat, may be coming from a need to downshift an overstimulated nervous system. In this case, the urge to eat is not something to be ignored, but eating may not necessarily be the best solution. Although it might be a quick fix, it will be temporary and cause side effects like weight gain. Better solutions may be found in allowing emotions to be expressed through breathwork, movement, or the other modalities we've discussed. But the very best solution is to make changes in your life so that you are not getting to the point of emotional overwhelm in the first place. So you see that the urge to eat is important, although eating may not be the long-term solution.

Since physical urges are very convincing, it is important to really get to know them intimately to be sure we are giving our bodies what they need rather than burying a bigger issue. As a free diver I have learned much about working with an overwhelming physical urge, the urge to take a breath. When working to increase breath holding time the first thing a diver needs to learn are the signs that the body truly needs oxygen. The first urges to breathe are not actually from a physical need for air but rather from the mind. The mind is unaccustomed to going such a long time without breathing and fear comes up. Fear produces the first urge to breathe. But the truth is that even though the urge to breathe is there, the body doesn't need air just yet. Anyone can hold their breath for a great deal of time beyond when the urge to breathe first arrives, if they are forced too. Somewhere into a breath hold the body starts swallowing, then slightly hiccuping, then the extremities start to tingle. Once the extremities tingle the need for oxygen is truly a physical need or will be quite soon. As a diver learns to recognize these biological signs, which come a long time after the mental/emotional urge to breathe, they can train their mind to stay calm and the urge to breathe will go away, sometimes for minutes. Training in breath holding is mostly about training the mind. In a similar way, we can explore our urges to eat. We can separate the mental from the physical and over time build a trusting relationship with our urges, knowing when to act and when to address emotions instead. When we get really good at this, it becomes really easy to trust our hunger, the same way we trust our bladder when it tells us it is time to find a bathroom.

Whenever we feel any urge, like the urge to eat, that urge holds important information for us. As in the case of free diving the initial urge to breathe comes from the mind and the emotion of fear. After practice I could easily sense the difference between fear and the need for air. So listening closely to our urges is the key to understanding when and how to act.

Let's say you're craving Oreos. There is an unopened family-sized package in the pantry. The craving is powerful. You suspect this isn't a physical need for food, but you feel paralyzed, afraid to twitch because the moment you move, your body is going to be floating across the room and into the pantry and your hands will be stuffing cookies into your face by their own accord. This is when you start body mapping. Where is this sensation in your body? What does it feel like? One of three things will happen. You may recognize an emotional signature and feel an urge to let that emotion out another way, like moving your body, having a conversation with someone, or getting a project done. Another possibility is that you recognize the emotional signature is not hunger but you don't know what it is, and you still want the Oreos. The last option is that you recognize the signature as true physical hunger, and you still want the Oreos. In either of the latter cases, the best thing to do is to eat the Oreos, very very mindfully. Notice every flavor, texture, and smell. Try to notice if you're becoming satiated. Whenever you are ready to stop eating, notice how you feel. Better, worse, or the same? Map your emotional state now. Map your physical state. Did you become satiated? Do you want something else now? Do you feel calmer or more out of control? How does your stomach feel? How is your energy level?

Continue noticing these things for the next several hours and even the next morning. If you did physically need a quick shot of sugar, you will feel awesome afterwards and can move on with your day. If, on the other hand, the Oreos were a temporary distraction from a real problem, you probably will eat more than you care to admit and feel worse both physically and mentally afterward. Either way, indulging the craving with great mindfulness is extremely important. Because if you had willpowered through it and just had a carrot stick instead, you would have learned nothing and just pushed the problem down the road. Mindfully letting a craving run its course is the only way that our bodies will teach our minds that eating Oreos is not a good solution to emotional overwhelm. By trusting the body and paying attention to its reaction we will have our answers. Trust and listen, listen and trust.

Chapter 18: Cultivate Awareness

If weight is like a check engine light alerting us to a deeper problem, then the very first thing we have to do is run diagnostics. Just like a mechanic, we want to take the car for a test drive and listen for any strange sounds. This listening process is critical and very enlightening. Let me give you a powerful tool for training your ear to hear what is going on below the hood.

We cannot change that which we are unaware of. Anyone who has dieted before is familiar with a food log. We won't be keeping a food log here! But we *will* keep a log about how you *feel* about what you ate. This is a simple journal. I encourage you to write in this journal a few times per week or more. You will write what you thought about what and how you ate it. (If you don't like to journal making a voice note in your phone is just as good.) If you ate a heavy dinner and noticed it made you feel tired, write about that. If you skipped breakfast and noticed you felt proud, write about that. If you wanted french fries but ordered a salad, write about why you did that. If you had dessert and felt guilty, write about that. Just keep in mind this is NOT a place to keep track of calories, macros, etc. It is a place to write about how you felt, physically and mentally, about the food choices you made that day.

Another important thing to note is how you were feeling when you first started to want to eat. Did you find yourself reaching for a snack in the car when you hit a traffic jam? Did you open your email, feel overwhelmed by a subject line, and get up for a trip to the vending machine? Notice if you make judgments about what you ate such as, "It was a good day," or "I ate way too much today." Eventually we want to be able to see what we ate as completely neutral. But don't beat yourself up if you have strong feelings about what and how you ate. Just make a note in the margin of "judgment thoughts" with an arrow to the relevant sentence. The point here is NOT to change ANYTHING but rather to become aware of what we are doing, feeling and thinking. Approach this activity as something fun, almost funny, getting to know the inner workings of your mind almost like you would get to know a fictional character in a movie. Try to be as honest with yourself as you can. The more you can admit your thoughts and feelings to yourself the quicker you can move beyond them. When you write something down, notice if it feels incomplete or a little off. See if there is something more you might be afraid to admit, even to yourself. When you notice yourself doing this, celebrate it, this is where you are really making progress!

So here are the things to write in your food journal:

1. How the things you ate made you feel physically.
2. How the things you ate made you feel mentally.
3. What you were feeling around the time you ate.
4. Any feelings of guilt or judgment (good or bad).
5. Any dieting behaviors you noticed yourself doing and why you think you did them.

And here are the things to avoid:

1. Writing down what and how much you ate.
2. Mentally calculating calories.
3. Doing this activity if you absolutely hate doing it and it feels like just another chore on your to-do list.

Lastly, if you just can't give up calorie counting or food logging, don't. You're not ready and there is nothing wrong with that. If you try to force yourself into something you're not ready for, it is going to backfire. Instead, just notice those urges to track and log and write about that. What is it about logging your foods (or any other dieting behavior) that feels good to you? Do you feel more in control? Does it give you a bit of peace if you can label a day as "good" or "bad"? Do you feel more empowered after having done it? The only wrong answer here is a dishonest answer. Remember, no one is judging you. The more honest you can be with yourself the faster you will experience complete food freedom.

Homework 10:

> Write in your food thoughts journal a few times per week over the next one to two months. You might want to buy a new journal or just create a new blank file on your phone or computer to keep all of these journals together.

Chapter 19: Conscious eating

Conscious eating is a way of nourishing the body that is aligned with three core principles: body trust, individual nutrition, and body kindness. Let's look at these one by one. Body trust is absolutely essential. Would you ever disallow yourself to act on the need to use the bathroom, citing not having drank enough water as a reason that you don't deserve to pee? Of course not! Because we have no reason to mistrust the need to pee. Likewise, once you've mastered the art of decoupling physical needs from other urges (or little "h" hunger from big "H" hunger) you can act on those physical needs with confidence. In other words, once you know it is true physical, little h hunger, eat! The idea is that the body knows what it needs for its optimum functioning. So when you feel physically hungry you can trust that you need to eat.

Learning to trust your hunger takes some time. Keep in mind there is no right or wrong, just good and better. The idea is to have fun and treat this like an art. You will know a sensation is true physical hunger (little "h") when eating what you are hungry for makes the sensation go away and you feel better after doing so. The steps for separating a physical need for food from a non-physical urge that is showing up as hunger are simple yet powerful.

1. Map the urge to eat in your body.
2. If you suspect the urge is actually for something else, do that instead. If the urge does not go away at that point, or you think it actually is true hunger, go to step three.
3. Eat whatever it is that you want to eat. But eat mindfully, paying attention to how the food looks, tastes, smells, and feels.
4. Pay attention to your satiety. Are you becoming satisfied or feeling more and more ravenous as you go?

5. Stop eating whenever you are ready to stop, no matter how much food that takes.
6. Consciously observe your physical body. Do you feel sick to your stomach? How is your energy? Does your head feel clear? etc.
7. Consciously observe your emotional state. Do you feel guilt? Do you still crave something but aren't sure what it is? Did the food actually help you feel better? Did the energy from the food translate into joy in your body?
8. Continue to be aware of your emotional and physical sensations over the course of the next hour and into the next morning.
9. Continue making these hunger maps until it is crystal clear what true physical hunger feels like in the body.

True physical hunger does have a lot of similarities in how it shows up for most people. Most people will feel a sense of emptiness in the low belly. They might feel or hear a rumbling in that area. Physical energy could be fading. Although low energy alone is not enough to signal hunger because low energy could also come from a lack of sleep or too much stress in life. Often people with low energy turn to food to compensate when in reality a few lifestyle changes could be a better solution.

When true physical hunger strikes, it is always satisfied by eating, eating enough, and eating what you are hungry for. So you will know it was true hunger if after having eaten, you feel satisfied. Refer to chapter fifteen on decoupling hunger to learn the signature of true physical hunger in the body. This is where body trust is so important. If you are truly hungry, eating is in the interest of your optimum physical health and your optimum weight. Your body knows how to heal a cut, recover from the flu and, if you're a person with ovaries, how to build a human. Trust that your body knows when to eat and feed itself when it is truly hungry! Not eating when you are truly hungry is going to lead to health issues and eventually even to weight gain.

Eating when you are hungry is only the first half of body trust. The second half is to stop when you are satisfied. Once again, we will need to create maps to know what it feels like to be satisfied. I do not use the word "full" here because your stomach does not need to be physically full in order to be satisfied. For example, a small piece of dark chocolate might be extremely satisfying while it certainly would not fill a stomach. So we will need to carefully map the feeling of satiety in order to know when to stop eating. Here is what that looks like.

The next time you notice that you are truly hungry, begin eating whatever it is that sounds good to you. Continue eating until you are ready to stop, even if that means eating an entire jar of peanut butter. You will pay close attention to what you think might be satiety, but don't stop eating until you want to stop. When you do stop, map how you feel. Do you feel energized and awake or sleepy and heavy? Do you want to move on with your day or lie down? Does your belly feel like it is pushing out or do you feel like your stomach has moved up under your ribs? Once again, there are some common signs that you may have eaten more than you needed for satiety: Heaviness, nausea, low energy, fatigue, and bloating. Just as in experiencing true hunger, understanding satiety will come with a period of trial and error. The idea is to continue eating until you want to stop, and each time pay attention before you stop, while you are stopping, and after you stop. If you are not sure what it feels like to be overly full, go ahead and do the opposite of the previous exercise. Once or twice, eat when you aren't truly hungry or eat more than you are hungry for. This is something interesting to try at Thanksgiving or a similar celebration. Go ahead, pig out. But then mindfully map out how it feels to be "stuffed." Once again, the only way for our minds to stop wanting more food than the body physically needs is to allow the mind to experience the physical discomfort of overeating. The body is trying to teach the mind. So get still and listen to it speak.

The first principle of conscious eating, body trust, can be summarized as follows. **Eat when you are hungry; stop**

when you are satisfied. This is not a rule, but rather a guideline. You can break it whenever you don't feel like following it. I stray from this principle at least a few times a year. When there is so much good food at a party or event that I couldn't possibly try it all without getting overly full, I enjoy it all. Then, just like drinking too much alcohol, I suffer the consequences of a food hangover, which was totally worth it, but if I am conscious about recognizing the consequences of my choices, I am unlikely to repeat those choices in the near future.

Individual nutrition is the second pillar of conscious eating. What works for one person is as unique as their fingerprints. There is no one way of eating that is best for everyone. Each person's body is their own best dietician. Most of us will have quite a lot of overlap on what makes our bodies operate optimally. But each of us will have large differences as well. Once again, we rely on the internal wisdom of the body to tell us what, when and how much to eat. There have been times in my life when a big protein filled breakfast has been super important. There have been other times when delaying breakfast for a few hours feels better than eating right away and still other times when grabbing a banana on the way out the door has felt just right. Feel free to ignore any supposed authority figure on the internet who says, "My way of eating is the best way of eating." There are no right or wrong ways of eating anymore, just what is optimal and subpar for *you* at this moment in time for *your* unique needs.

We can summarize this principle as follows: **eat what you are hungry for**. This guideline, again, will need to be examined with great mindfulness. On the surface you may think that eating whatever you want will mean living on cheesecake and potato chips. And if that is what sounds good to you then you definitely should eat cheesecake and potato chips. And while doing so you will need to apply the ideas of eating mindfully and mapping the way these foods make you feel, physically and mentally. Trust your body. It won't take long before it is craving a salad!

Some of you who have dieted, restricted, cut out entire food groups or dropped significantly lower than your healthiest weight will absolutely need to eat highly palpable foods for a period of time. You might even eat them incredibly mindfully and still be unable to notice these foods causing the body any distress. In that case, keep eating them, mindfully. If you are truly physically hungry, and you are truly hungry for cookies, eat as many cookies as you want to eat until you feel satisfied. And of course, notice how the cookies taste, smell, and feel. Notice how you feel before, during, and after.

When I first fired the food police and fully embraced this second guideline of eating whatever I was hungry for, I had a lot of lost time to make up for. I wasn't underweight because I had already been practicing the first guideline of conscious eating (eating when I was hungry and stopping when I was satisfied) for over a year. But I was still limiting my foods to what felt safe. I had been living with restrictive food rules for almost twenty years at that point. It was Christmas time, and I was staying with my parents when I finally decided to let myself eat what I was hungry for. My mom loves to bake. I wanted nothing but her homemade cookies and so that is what I ate for three weeks straight. When January hit and I returned home, I asked my mom for the recipe for her Monster Cookies. I must have made five or six triple batches that month. Those cookies made up about 75% of my diet for about a month. Then suddenly a switch flipped. The cookies just didn't sound good anymore. Just like that they were too sweet for me. The last five cookies sat in the fridge for two months before I finally threw them out. Did I gain weight? You betcha! Was it really challenging to see myself getting bigger? Absolutely. And then I promptly lost the weight, plus a lot more, without even trying, faster than I had ever been able to lose weight on any diet, and I've kept it off for many years. I still eat Monster Cookies here and there. But now I can eat one or two when they sound good and later forget about them for months.

From here on out whatever sounds good when you are hungry is absolutely the best choice for you, even if it's

Monster Cookies. Trust that your body needs it and that it will tell you when it needs something else. Then listen. How did that food make you feel? Your body will tell you if it was the best choice or not. Some foods take longer than others to get the hang of. Specifically sweet, salty, and oily foods. Many food companies have engineered their food in a way that makes it very hard to hear the distress of our bodies over the fantastic flavor of the food. These foods, if they are negatively affecting your body, will take a lot of practice before you definitely don't want to eat them based on want-power alone. And that is perfectly fine. Remember, no more willpower. If you want it, have it. Just pay attention! If you feel conflicted, like you really want a food, but you feel like that particular food isn't optimal for your health, then those are the moments you want to eat the most slowly with the most mindfulness. Again, want-power only. Eventually you will hear your body protesting and foods that no longer serve you will no longer sound appetizing to you.

Just today I ate a highly processed chocolate chip cookie. My husband is a cookie monster and always keeps them in the house. When we first started living together, I was eating one or two daily. But they started to leave me feeling a little let down, like I didn't get my money's worth. One day I looked at them and they sorta looked good but then I thought about how they had been leaving me wanting recently and decided to have a piece of dark chocolate instead. Now, every couple of weeks they look good again. So I have one. And every time I do, I am disappointed. "Nope, not that great." I never thought I'd get to this point with sweets, but it is happening and it will happen for you too!

The final core principle is body kindness. If you have ever cared for a small child whom you love, then you know exactly what this means already. If the child says he is hungry, you don't question him, you feed him. The choice of what to feed him is made by a quick calculation involving what is available, what you have time to prepare, what is nutritious, and what he is willing to eat. You quickly assess all these variables and then choose a meal for the child. If he wants a food that you know is not nutritious for him you occasionally say yes, occasionally say no, and occasionally say yes but only after he's eaten his veggies. The only reason you are saying no to him is because he isn't old enough to be able to associate a temper tantrum with Halloween candy. But you can, so you guide him with love.

He doesn't understand mindful eating and the idea of paying attention to the consequences of his food choices, so you help him with those choices. You say yes sometimes because you want him to be a part of a birthday party. Because feeling left out would be worse for him than the sugar rush. Or maybe you say yes because you simply want to see a big smile on his face. You are always weighing the pros and cons and making the best decisions for him out of love. And it isn't just with food. You are deciding between letting him stay up to enjoy a book or making him turn the lights out. You make sure you pack all the things you need when you leave the house so that he won't be uncomfortable. You spend money to buy him the things he needs. Basically, you treat him and his physical needs with kindness and respect. Somehow, we never learned to do the same for ourselves. But that is exactly what principle three says: **respect the needs of your body**.

This guideline is about nourishing your body in all the ways it needs nourishing: with food, with sleep, with exercise, with routine, with breathing, with resting, with recreation, with sex, with artistic expression, with physical touch, and anything else you feel the body craves. It is about giving your body the very best that you can give it based on what is available to you. It might seem strange to have this principle in the conscious eating section since it is about more than just food. But if we are not taking care of all of the needs of the body, they will often spill over into an increased appetite for food. For example, I always feel hungry when I'm woken early from a nap I really needed. All of the physical needs of the body are interrelated so respecting them all is critical when eating for optimal health and weight.

These are the only three guidelines you will need for the rest of your life. Let's review the conscious eating guidelines.

1. **Eat when you are hungry; stop when you are satisfied.**
2. **Eat what you are hungry for.**
3. **Respect the needs of your body.**

Homework 11:
1. Postpone one meal or snack this week at a time when you're pretty sure you are physically hungry. Map what hunger feels like in your body and write it down.
2. Purposely overeat at one meal or snack this week. Map what being overly full feels like in your body and write it down.
3. Eat at least one food you normally would not allow. Be sure you are hungry and hungry for that food at the same time. Then eat the food mindfully, paying attention to flavor, texture, and smell. Notice any cravings to eat beyond the point of satiety. If you do overeat, don't worry, just notice how it makes you feel. Whether you overeat or not, notice how you feel immediately afterwards, an hour later, and the next morning.
4. Journal/thought/voice note question. At the end of the day ask yourself, "Where did I push myself or restrict myself in a way that wasn't respectful toward the desires of my body?"

Chapter 20: Conscious Movement

Our bodies are designed to be used. Only in recent history have humans had the ability to sit for more waking hours than not while still providing for our physical needs. Even just a couple of generations ago humans still spent most of their waking hours up and about, pushing, pulling, bending, lifting, walking, climbing, carrying, and standing. In modern western culture, especially post-COVID-19, it is completely possible to wake up, grab your computer, and never leave your bed except to grab a food delivery from the front door. Obviously, this is going to have a big effect on a person's health.

On the other hand there is a "fitness" culture evolving that is very disturbing. Now many of us are "too strong for weak days" or rather, "too weak to admit we need rest." There are "fitness" modeling competitions where people starve themselves for weeks in order for their muscles to show more prominently. We love our "boot camp" classes. Did you know a real boot camp is a time when young, head-strong people are broken into submission to an authority? High intensity interval training instructors tell their students to push until they feel like they "are going to die." Some types of hot yoga classes do not allow students to leave the room even if they worry they will pass out. Whatever all of this is about, it certainly isn't kind. This "no pain, no gain" mentality is outdated and needs an upgrade. This is where conscious movement comes in. Conscious movement is based on three core principles: stewardship, joy and respect. Let's take a look at each one. And obviously, before you start any exercise program, check with your doctor!

To be a steward is to be a caretaker. A steward is in charge of using the resources of an entity and providing for that entity's needs. Conscious movement asks us to be the stewards of our own bodies. Bodies need to be moved. It is a basic core need of every body to move. So the first conscious movement guideline is to *move intentionally every day*. Some days this will literally be just shaking and wiggling your body to clear the lymphatic system. When I am seriously ill, this is pretty much what I can handle. Some days this will be five minutes of gentle stretching or a walk around the block or taking the stairs an extra two flights or parking at the far side of the parking lot. If movement is new to you and this feels like a lot, then trust that it is enough. Some days this might be an hour or more of lifting weights or even a bootcamp style class if that is what feels good to you. The idea, similar to conscious eating, is to trust your body. Check in before, during, and after the movement. Do what feels empowering, compassionate, and kind for your body.

The next principle is *joy,* and its corresponding guideline is *do movement that brings you joy*. So if you really love CrossFit then by all means go for it. But if you are counting down the minutes until the end of class, just get your stuff and go home early. Conscious movement asks you to find an activity that brings you joy and to do that more days than not. Often this is a sport or a class such as tennis, golf, surfing, yoga, or dance. Find a form of movement that you enjoy that is both mentally stimulating and physically challenging and then do it as often as is fun for you. When I found surfing, I fell in love with it. Suddenly surfing became the reason to do yoga, to work on my cardio, or to get stronger legs. Before surfing I would force myself to do these exercises because it seemed like that is what I needed to do in order to look good and be healthy. It took willpower. After I found surfing, I was motivated to stretch so that I could surf again the next day without pain. I was motivated to do cardio so that I could surf for longer sessions without fatiguing. I was motivated to go to the gym so I could do stronger maneuvers on my surfboard. It was a game changer. This is *Joyful Movement*. If you haven't found your surfing yet, keep looking! Try classes, leagues, and clubs until the right thing calls to you. And if you're a person who really dislikes exercise then remember to really tune into how you are feeling before, during, and after. Find a form of movement that feels good in your body. When it feels good, you'll stick to it. At first it might seem challenging because you aren't used to it. Start small. Even vacuuming the house once a day may be enough to challenge you. But really pay attention to how your stamina, energy, libido, mood, and overall motivation is increasing. You will start to see positive changes in the way you are feeling if you practice looking for them. Increase duration, frequency, and intensity when it feels right.

The third principle, respect, has to do with finding the right amount of movement. I will summarize this in the following guideline: *find the "Goldilocks Zone."* The Goldilocks Zone comes from the classic children's story where the little girl, Goldilocks, wanders into the home of three bears. She finds the baby's porridge too cold, the papa's porridge too hot and the mama's porridge just right.

In exercise, the Goldilocks zone represents the place where your body is being challenged just the right amount. Someone who is unaccustomed to exercise will have a very different Goldilocks zone than a professional athlete. Only you know when you are in this zone. You will feel challenged but not depleted. You will feel some physical discomfort but no pain. You will feel stronger after a few days rather than sick, tired, injured, or no change at all. Not enough movement will mean poor digestion, muscle stiffness, poor sleep, moodiness, hormonal imbalances, lethargy, and weakness. Too much movement also will result in poor sleep, moodiness, hormonal imbalances, illness, and lethargy, as well as pain and injury. On the other hand, exercise in the Goldilocks zone will result in better sleep, balanced hormones, increased overall energy (although it might dip for a couple of hours afterward), increased muscle tone and stamina, and improved digestion. You may feel a bit sore for a day or two, but it won't be to the point of interfering with normal daily activities. Some soreness is a good thing. For some of you, finding the Goldilocks zone will mean cutting back on the intensity of your movement and for others this will mean stepping it up. Are you an overachiever? Do you always need a project? Do you prioritize growth? Then chances are you may have a tendency to overdo it with regard to the intensity of your workouts. For you go-getters, I suggest tapering back a bit. On the other hand if you are a professional relaxer, love your down time, and prioritize rest then chances are you might need to step it up a little when it comes to exercising.

Let's summarize the three conscious movement guidelines:
1. **Move intentionally every day.**
2. **Do movement that brings you joy.**
3. **Find the Goldilocks Zone.**

Remember, you are your best personal trainer. No one knows your body as well as you will when you listen to it. Doing movement mindfully is the key here. Here are some questions to improve mindfulness and help you to act on your own biofeedback.

Before you start, ask yourself:
- How is my energy level?
- Do I feel pain or soreness anywhere?
- What kind of movement sounds good to me today?

During the movement, ask yourself:
- Am I enjoying this or at least seeing the benefit in doing it?
- Is this causing me pain?
- Do I feel challenged?
- Is this depleting me or making me stronger?

Immediately after the movement, ask yourself:
- Do I feel so tired that I need a nap?
- Do I feel a nice endorphin boost?
- Was that a kind thing to do to my body?
- Was that fun?

Over the next forty-eight hours, ask yourself:
- On a scale of 1-10 how sore am I? (1=not at all, 5=just right 10=serious pain)
- Did the movement seem to improve my sleep?
- Do I feel run down?

- Do I feel ready to repeat that or would a different form of movement (possibly involving different muscle groups) feel better?

Over a span of one to two months ask:

- Am I still loving this style of movement?
- Am I getting stronger?
- How is my sleep?
- How is my overall energy and stamina?
- Am I getting sick or injured?

The last point we need to discuss is the matter of priorities. I often hear, "But I don't have time to work out!" There is enough time in your day for anything you prioritize. When you do not prioritize movement, your body suffers. When the body is suffering, we are less effective in the workplace. We are more tired, less creative, and our ability to collaborate suffers. When the body is suffering, so too are our families. We snap at the kids, neglect our partners, and project a negative energy about the house. Prioritizing movement is truly a shortcut to be more successful in everything else that is important to us. Here are a few ideas to help you prioritize movement. If you have little kids at home, try signing up for mommy-and-me classes or try using your toddler as an alternative to hand weights during body weight exercises. If you work and parent full time, try doing home workouts to save time driving to classes or gyms, such as videos, gardening, yardwork, or body weight exercises. Get the kids involved if they are into it. Play a sport with them or take them with you to age-appropriate classes. You might join a rock-climbing gym, go roller skating, or take a bike ride together on the weekends when your schedule has a bit of family time already blocked out. Not only will you be doing valuable movement and spending quality time with your children, but you will also be modeling for them the importance of having fun while moving the body. And if your job is so demanding that you are working every waking hour, stop. I promise, that is not the most effective way to accomplish your work goals. Even Einstein took breaks to ride his bike in order to improve his problem-solving ability. Schedule two half-hour breaks into your day to get outside and move around. Try it for a week and I promise you'll be amazed at how much more you can get done!

Homework 12:
1. Evaluate your current movement habits. Are you stewarding your body by moving every day? Do you love your workout schedule? Are you over or under training?
2. If you don't already have a movement routine that you love, find one! Sign up for a class, join a club, or buy the equipment you need for a new sport or hobby. After giving it a fair chance, if you don't love it, try something else until you find what you do love!
3. If you do have a movement routine that you already love, evaluate if you need to do more or cut back. Then take action to do so right away!

Chapter 21: Intentional Weight Loss

You may have heard of something called the Set Point Theory which postulates that each of us has a "healthiest" weight for our unique body. I like to talk about something similar which I call "Optimum Weight" or the weight at which your body, mind, emotions, and spirit function optimally. You will know you are at your optimal weight when you are eating by the Conscious Eating guidelines and your weight never varies by more than a few pounds in either direction.

With optimal weight, a body holds a certain amount of weight that is optimal for a time period, but optimal weight changes when lifestyle or circumstances change. For example, someone who is stressed and overworked may need extra weight to help balance cortisol levels. Someone going through menopause may need extra weight while the body establishes equilibrium with reduced estrogen. Someone recovering from an eating disorder may need extra weight until the body learns there is no risk of famine anymore. In those cases, being "overweight" may actually be the healthiest condition for the body as it deals with physical, mental, emotional, and spiritual challenges. But once the outside circumstances change (stress is reduced, hormones are balanced, or the eating disorder has completely healed), then the body is able to find a new "optimal weight." This is why focusing on weight loss isn't useful. The body knows what it needs and when we address all the underlying causes of excess weight, the weight falls off naturally, almost like a side effect. So the very best way to lose weight is to focus on changing the circumstances that contribute to being at your optimal weight.

That being said, in addition to mental, spiritual, and emotional reasons a body might be holding extra weight, there are also physical reasons a body might be holding extra weight which are related to what we eat and how we move. There is some time-tested, non-fad advice on how to care for our bodies, physically, in order to reach optimal weight. Before I get into these Intentional Weight Loss Strategies, let's review the no-no's.

1. Never restrict your calories. If you are hungry, eat. (Review the difference between little "h" and big "H" hunger if necessary.)
2. Never restrict certain foods. If you want to eat it, eat it! (Review the mindful eating steps. Remember, eventually you won't even want foods that are unhealthy for you.)
3. Do not weigh yourself. (Weight will fluctuate up and down. This is a journey not a sprint. This is about health, not a number on a scale.)
4. Enjoy the journey. If it sucks, don't do it. Fitness first, joy ALWAYS!

Now that we know what *not* to do, let's take a look at these time-tested Intentional Weight Loss Strategies.

1. *Focus on eating more veggies.*

This isn't about cutting anything out but rather adding in. You don't have to swap fries for a salad if you truly want the fries. Just order the salad too and have both! Stock your house with the veggies you like the most. Consider pre-chopping them to have them convenient for cooking and snacking. Frozen veggies are a great way to quickly add veggies to almost any home cooked meal. Add a handful of leafy greens to a smoothie. Eat veggies you like as often as you can.

2. *Wait for the "good" kind of hungry.*

Wait to eat meals until your body really needs it. Again, this should not take willpower. You should be able to enjoy the hunger because the food tastes better when you wait and you feel so much more energized after eating, as opposed to eating too soon and feeling tired and sluggish. I love the feeling I get after surfing for a couple of hours. I am ravenous and everything tastes so good. This is what I'm talking about when I say the good kind of hungry. Sometimes I get very hungry before dinner time and have a heavy snack. Then an hour later when I sit down to dinner, I end up eating just because the food is there. This makes me feel heavy and tired. Some people will feel really good by letting their digestive system have a rest for a couple of extra hours each day. I recommend doing this only if you can enjoy this "good" kind of hunger and feel the benefits it is bringing to your body. If it feels hard and is taking willpower, rest assured this is hurting rather than helping and skip it. Finding the good kind of hungry will take a bit of practice. You will feel it most strongly after intense exercise.

Once you've learned to feel this "good" hunger and enjoy it then you can try something I call Delayed Eating. This technique is for those who are advanced in their attunement to their bodies only. If you are just beginning to work with body maps and emotional signatures, I suggest you wait until you become adept at quickly noticing subtle sensations before you try this. Delayed Eating is like intermittent fasting but much gentler on the body and driven only by want-power because it feels good. This should be the opposite of depriving. Here are the steps to Delayed Eating:

1. Try waiting to eat breakfast until the "good kind of hungry" strikes.

2. You might try not snacking after dinner, so you wake up hungry or delaying breakfast for about fifteen minutes until you feel the "good kind of hungry."

3. If it feels good, continue pushing breakfast back a few minutes per week.

4. IF IT FEELS GOOD, you can exercise in the morning before you've had a meal.

5. IF IT FEELS GOOD, you can space out dinner and breakfast by twelve or more hours.

Delayed Eating is a powerful weight loss tool because it allows your digestive system to have time to recover between meals. It is important to remember that this should feel good. You should be able to feel your improved digestion and use that as a motivating factor. In other words, this whole tool is based on body kindness not self-deprivation or punishment. But there are two things you need to be extremely conscious of. First, are you being triggered? Do you find yourself falling back into old dieting behaviors? Are you checking your weight? Using coffee or other appetite suppressants? Are you tempted to count your calories? If so, discontinue Delayed Eating immediately. Secondly, Delayed Eating needs to honor changing hormone levels, especially for women. During ovulation Delayed Eating might feel natural and energizing. While just prior to menstruation it may feel depleting and difficult. Menopause is another time when Delayed Eating may be all wrong for the body. Again, I cannot stress enough, if it doesn't feel good then it isn't helping you to lose weight. Feel free to skip or abbreviate Delayed Eating any time it doesn't feel good.

3. *Be extra mindful when eating certain foods.*

There are foods that are engineered by food scientists to override our internal signaling system to make us want more and more. There are other foods that are designed by nature to make us want more and more because those foods helped us survive when periods of famine were common in our early evolution. The increasing accessibility of these foods within the last one hundred years hasn't allowed the natural signaling system to catch up. So even after you get really good at the conscious eating principles certain foods are going to take extra effort to keep consumption levels in check for optimum health. These foods are:

- Sugar and sugar alternatives
- Processed/packaged foods
- Fried foods

- Processed grains (especially ones with added fat or sugar such as baked goods)
- Alcohol

Never in a million years am I saying these foods should be cut out of your diet. Absolutely not. I'm not even suggesting you limit or restrict yourself with these foods. The idea is that if you want to eat this food do so with great mindfulness (review the conscious eating questions if you need). If these foods are not serving the body toward optimum health, the body will indeed signal you through sensations, albeit muffled sensations. This is why it is very important to listen up. When you can feel the body having a bad reaction you will no longer want to eat that particular food. For example I used to use a lot of monk fruit sweetener until I noticed it was giving me a lot of gas. Now whenever a package says, "Sweetened with Monk Fruit," I promptly put it back on the shelf, no willpower necessary! As with anything worth doing, this is a process, and it will take practice. There is no need to set high standards here. Little by little is how this is done. It took me five years before I could feel my body reacting poorly to excess cookies and baked goods. Once I finally heard it my "sugar addiction" slowly faded away.

A Note on Sugar: Merriam-Webster defines an addition as a compulsive, chronic, physiological or psychological need for a habit-forming substance, behavior, or activity having harmful physical, psychological, or social effects and typically causing well-defined symptoms (such as anxiety, irritability, tremors, or nausea) upon withdrawal or abstinence. *So, if you feel it is hurting you and yet you still feel a compulsion to do it, then it is an addiction. For some people, sugar (and other foods) qualify as an addition. Sugar certainly did for me. When I got my cancer diagnosis my doctor urged me to cut out all sugar. It was really hard! I didn't want to eat sugar yet I still did it. Plus, it was hurting me. I was addicted. By using the Conscious Eating Principles, sitting with my discomfort and being both mindful and gentle with myself I was able to break the addiction. It took a long time! At first I tried to go cold turkey but soon found myself binging on fruit. I knew I had to be gentler and respect the limits of my body. There was trial and error involved. In the end, what worked was to follow my intuition and let desire lead the way. I began to feel a difference between a compulsion to eat sugar and a desire be healthy. Little by little, over the course of many months I was able to adjust to a diet lower in sugar without feeling like I was depriving myself of something I really wanted. I can trust my body. Since the addiction is gone, if I feel the urge to have sugar I know it is coming from a physiological need rather than a dependence. This is a very tricky issues and the lines get blurry. My best advice is to take it slow, don't force anything and be honest with yourself as much as possible. Does your relationship with sugar feel healthy or does it feel like sugar holds all the power? Is sugar truly hurting you or is adding to the enjoyment of life? Remember, only you can really know the answer to this.*

4.   *Do movement that temporarily spikes the heart rate.*

Remember to first adhere to the conscious movement guidelines. You must enjoy the movement and it must not be too taxing on the body. That being said, there are many forms of movement that spike the heart rate for a short time, and they don't have to be brutal. This type of movement is fantastic for regulating hormones and helping the body to use excess fat stores. Here are some examples:

- Sports like soccer, basketball, softball, and surfing.
- Activities like frisbee, catch, or wrestling with kids.
- Classes like dance, boot camp, or HIIT (Remember not to overdo it with these and to only do it if you enjoy it!)
- Incorporate "sprint" intervals into walks, bikes, paddle boarding, or swimming.

This type of heart rate spiking movement should only be done two to three times per week at most especially if you are really pushing. If you overdo it here, the body will feel depleted and will ask you for highly palatable food in order to recover, and lots of it! This is a case where more is not better and there is a point of dimensioning returns. Balance can be found by listening to the body. Also recognize that your menstrual cycle will affect your energy levels so feel free to skip a workout (or three) when you need extra rest. Remember that the very best results can be achieved by working with your body rather than against it. Yes, it may take a little longer to get to your goals, but not only will the process be way more fun, the results will stick around for good!

5.   *Build Muscle*

Muscle keeps the metabolism high and helps the body through hormonal changes. You will know you are building muscle if you are a little sore the next day. (The older you are the longer it will take to feel sore so don't be surprised if it takes forty-eight hours or more before you feel it). If you aren't sore at all, then you can go a little harder; if you are very sore or in pain, then you need to cut back. Find a form of exercise that you ENJOY that builds muscles. Here are some great options.
- Vinyasa Yoga
- Pilates
- Weightlifting
- Swimming
- Body weight workouts
- TRX

Remember to check with your doctor before starting any exercise program and always follow the movement guidelines first. If it isn't fun, try something else. If it leaves you overly sore and depleted, cut back on either frequency, intensity, or duration (do it less often per week, do fewer reps or lighter weights, or do it for less time).

So let's summarize the Intentional Weight Loss Strategies:

1. Focus on eating more veggies.
2. Wait for the "good" kind of hungry.
3. Be extra mindful when eating certain foods.
4. Do movement that temporarily spikes the heart rate.
5. Build muscle.

Homework 13:

> If you think you NEED to lose weight (for health reasons) make an appointment to discuss with your doctor if you are truly experiencing health issues due to your weight. If you NEED to lose weight for your HEALTH and you have permission from your doctor, start very slowly trying only one of the strategies above. Master that strategy before adding in another one. ALWAYS with JOY. Never power through it!

> If you just want to lose a few pounds or your doctor says you are already at a healthy weight, then I urge you to simply stick to the Conscious Eating Guidelines and the Conscious Movement Guidelines. Those guidelines will be enough to guide you to a healthy, happy, balanced body.

Chapter 22: Meal Planning

Part of the draw of a diet is the ease of having someone else tell you what to do. It is all laid out for you in bullet points. Good little girls love rules. It makes us feel safe. Somewhere in early childhood we realized that if we follow the rules, then we will be liked. And if we are liked then we will get our needs met; we will be safe. But the truth is no one is the authority on how to live your life except you and following someone else's rules will always lead to burn out, eventually.

I had a calculus teacher who took questions on homework problems for the first half hour of class. If someone asked, "How do you do number nine?" he wouldn't even respond. But if someone asked, "I tried number nine. I got to the point where I integrated by parts twice but I'm not sure how to solve for the unknown interval. What do I do with the constant factor?" then he would leap into action at the whiteboard.

Lists of what and when to eat are quite like the professor doing the homework for the students. You don't learn anything and when it comes to test time, you're going to fail. So rather than giving you meal plans I prefer to help you understand how to meal plan. In the long run, meal planning ahead of time doesn't work for most people. But having a basic working knowledge of sound, time tested nutritional information can help you to make healthy choices on the go. Most people like to have a set breakfast that they eat on most days. So that is an easy one to pre-plan. If you pack a lunch to bring to work, then this is another time when you might be able to pre-plan what you will eat. But be sure to leave plenty of flexibility if you want to change your mind. There should be zero guilt here!

So here they are, the meal planning guidelines:

1. Follow the Conscious Eating Guidelines first and foremost. Don't worry if your meal choices don't

include everything I'm about to list. The number one thing is that you are eating when you are hungry, stopping when you are satisfied, eating what you are hungry for, and respecting the needs of your body. The Conscious Eating Guidelines trump all the other guidelines. For example, if you are hungry and your only options are soda crackers or red Jell-O, just eat whatever one sounds better and move on with your day. You can get something more nourishing when it becomes available.

2. Include living food. We are talking about fruits and veggies, nuts and seeds, raw or cooked. Ideally this is the majority of the food on your plate. Try to eat a variety of colors throughout the week. Fruits and veggies are loaded with the micronutrients we need, vitamins and minerals. It is fine to take a multivitamin, but micronutrients are much better absorbed when they come straight from your food.

3. Include fiber. If you followed guideline number two, then you automatically followed this guideline since living foods are loaded with fiber. Fiber helps with satiety and helps eliminate toxins.

4. In a single meal or snack include at least two of the following macronutrients: Carbohydrates, fat, or protein. In a single day be sure to include all three. You can read all over the internet about how much of each type of macronutrient you should have, and it will often conflict. Remember you are your best dietician. Listen to the needs of your body. Any science that says you shouldn't eat any carbs or another macronutrient should be evaluated with caution. Keto is a huge craze at the time of the publishing of this book. Rest assured, just like the low-fat craze of the nineties, once the long-term effects have been studied, the science will show Keto is neither healthy nor effective for long term weight loss. Some people, such as athletes, may feel better with lower fat and higher carbohydrate meals. This will provide quick energy without feeling heavy. Other

more sedentary people will require fewer carbohydrates and more fat to keep their brains active in mentally demanding careers. Whatever the case, eliminating an entire food group is generally not a good idea. But the real jury is your body and its reaction toward your diet. Let your body guide the way!

5. Drink mostly water. Drink sixty-four ounces or more of clean water daily.

6. You can eat five small meals, three moderate meals and two snacks, three large meals, two extra-large meals or just graze all day long. Whatever you do, follow the Conscious Eating Guidelines and evaluate how it works for your body. Modify as necessary.

7. Whenever possible, choose organic foods or at least non-GMO foods (organic automatically means non-GMO). Choose foods that have no ingredients (such as an apple) or very few ingredients. Choose foods that do not have artificial flavors, colors, or preservatives. That being said, if you really want the bag of BBQ potato chips filled with GMOs, preservatives, and artificial colors and flavors, go for it! Without any guilt, be mindful of how it makes you feel.

8. Check labels for added sugar. I'm not saying not to eat these foods. Simply become aware of how much added sugar you are eating so you can notice how it feels in your body. If it doesn't feel good, you will naturally want to ditch it. But we can't do that if we are not aware.

Let me stress, I do not follow the above meal planning guidelines at every meal, and I don't suggest you do either, unless you really want to. I eat plenty of meals without many veggies or with conventional ingredients or added sugar. I would say I follow these guidelines about 80% of the time. That is what works for me. If these guidelines feel like a big stretch, then just pick one of them that sounds good to you and start there. Or instead of following them 100% or even 80% of the time, just shoot for sixty/forty.

Homework 14:

Write your own meal plans. Design a day of ideal eating FOR YOU. The first consideration should be what sounds good to you. Follow the above guidelines as much or little as you want. Keep in mind you might be designing five small meals or just two extra-large meals, whatever works for you. Then be aware how you feel when implementing your plan. Do you want to eat it? Does something else sound better? Did you change your mind? Was it enough food to satisfy you? Did you enjoy eating it? Challenge yourself to abandon ship halfway through the day if you aren't loving the plan.

Chapter 23: Hormones and Aging

Bodies age. This is a fact we cannot avoid. These days celebrities spend ridiculous amounts of money and go through insanely invasive procedures in order to hide their age. But in the long run this isn't doing anyone any good. We will all get old. We will all die. As a person living with stage IV cancer, this topic is near and dear to my heart.

Every couple of weeks now I am faced with the inability to do something that I used to be able to do with ease. For most of my life I felt that I was expanding, growing, and producing. And then, like all people eventually do, I came face to face with the other side of expansion: contraction. This phase is about dying, but not just physically. It is the death of ego, of clinging, and of trying. Many things are dying away for me: my need for people to like me, my need to censor myself, my impatience, and intolerance. In this phase I am finally able to give myself permission to rest, enjoy, celebrate, and authentically express myself. Likewise, I am able to give the people around me the ability to be themselves without judgment from me. I feel more graceful, less harsh, more fluid, and less contained. It is truly a wonderful journey for which I am very grateful, even though I would not have chosen it.

We will all move into the contraction phase soon or later. We have a choice to make: will we be dragged into contraction kicking and screaming and Botoxing and hormone replacing or will we flow with the river of life wherever it might take us? Have you ever seen an elderly woman with wrinkles and white hair who immediately struck you as absolutely gorgeous? When you see her, you will know. Even though her face is wrinkled, it is soft. Even though her hair is white, it is lush. She has a grace and ease about her that makes you want to sit down and stay a while. There is wisdom under her words. She doesn't try to teach unless she is asked directly for her opinion. And even then, she will often talk around a subject, leaving room for the listener to find their own way. You wonder if she knows more about you than you know of yourself because she seems to see right through you. It feels as if she is both quiet and larger than life. She is radiant. She is majestic. Somehow, without clinging to youth, she has become more beautiful than ever before. We all have the ability to be this woman with age.

In mythology there are three female archetypes, the Maiden, the Mother, and the Crone. The word crone has quite negative connotations in modern culture. A sour, shriveled up, ugly woman might come to mind. But there is a movement to reclaim this word in current fourth-wave feminism. The Crone represents the phase in a woman's life where her focus has turned inward. It is a time for growing in wisdom and intuition. In cultures unlike our youth-obsessed culture, the crone represents the medicine woman, the elder, and the wise woman.

Once, while traveling in a remote fishing village in Mexico, I was scolded by a handsome young man in his twenties. I had just walked into his family's palapa and breezed right by a fat old woman sitting silently in an oversized chair with a cat in her lap, without so much as a nod in her direction. "You didn't greet my grandmother," he said, glaring at me. Even though I walked less than five feet from her, my brain honestly hadn't registered her presence. So trained are we in modern western culture to disregard the elderly.

Here is the truth about hormonal changes, they change a woman's physical appearance. Because of the drop in estrogen, the body is less likely to store fat in the breast and hips and more likely to store it in the belly. Not only that, but it also becomes more difficult to maintain muscle tone which makes it harder to maintain lean body mass. Meaning the average woman will gain weight. Additionally, since estrogen is what keeps everything supple in the body, not only will skin start to look dryer and saggier, but joints will also start to ache making exercise increasingly difficult. Of course there are many people ready to sell you solutions to these "problems." But what if none of these were problems in the first place? What if aging is exactly what needs to happen to move us into the best versions of ourselves? What if nature, in all its wisdom, didn't screw up when it designed women to go through menopause? What if all of this is happening *for* us rather than *to* us?

Of course there is no shame in heading to your local medi-spa, plastic surgeon, or hormone replacement doctor to help maintain some of your devolving youthfulness. Women for ages have gone to great lengths to embellish their natural beauty. Evidence of jewelry, makeup, and hair pieces goes back to prehistoric times. Women have always given great energy to the way they dressed from the time people began to clothe themselves. This is completely natural. And so too it is natural that as the options for maintaining a youthful appearance have increased that we would want to engage in using those options. I ask one simple question: What is the origin of your desire to enhance your appearance? Is it from lack or from love? When you go to get your gray hair colored do you feel more like a teenager trying desperately to cover a pimple with makeup or a queen adorning herself with jewels?

I raise the question of lack versus love because anything done from a lack mentality will never satisfy us even if it does achieve the desired result. Once the frown lines are Botoxed away, there will be lips in need of fillers. Once the lips are filled, there will be a cheek in need of microneedling. Unless you have endless money, endless time, and an endless pain tolerance, it will never end.

As a person who had to undergo surgical menopause at the age of thirty-eight as a life saving measure, without the option for hormone replacement therapy, I want to impart to you that aging is wonderful. And it sucks. But it is also wonderful. It is never easy to face change, but always necessary, and in this case, also good. The softening of rough edges, the strengthening of boundaries, the deepening of intuition, it is all magical. And it only happens through allowing. So we can age and fight it, or we can age and learn from it. Either way you will be beautiful, it's just a matter of outward vs inward beauty. Which do you prefer? For me that is an easy decision, but it would not have been even ten years ago. Just like everything else I have advocated in this book, you will be ready when you are ready. Let go a little at a time and receive a little at a time or let it all go and receive it all, it really doesn't matter. Go inward and rely on your intuition.

I definitely want to share with you some strategies for maintaining a strong, functional body as you age. While it is true that you may have to let go of a competitive mentality, forcing your body to be the best, it is also true that maintaining a healthy body composition will be helpful for overall health and energy. There are two strategies I will provide here.

1. *Do weight bearing exercise.*
The idea is to maintain muscle tone as much as possible. The very best activity here is weightlifting. Of course this should always follow the conscious movement guidelines, it should be fun, and done within the Goldilocks Zone. If weights aren't your thing, Pilates or other body weight exercises are also good options. Swimming is a wonderful way to build lean muscle. But any exercise is going to be better than no exercise. The best form of exercise is the one that you enjoy and will stick to, so make that your top priority here.

If you choose to lift weights, after doctor approval, I highly suggest doing a couple of sessions with a personal trainer if weights are new to you. Keep in mind trainers are often young and strong. They may not understand the challenges of beginning a lifting practice as an older adult. You want them to show you how to use the equipment safely and how to maintain a good form. But you may have to firmly express yourself when you are tired and do not wish to continue with a particular exercise. Don't let anyone push you around even if they are the "expert." The truth is that you are the expert on your body. Here are my best practices for lifting to build lean muscle mass.

- Start with very low weight.

- If you get to the eighth repetition and still feel very little fatigue, you can increase the weight on the next set. If the weight is starting to get hard to lift before the eighth rep, then it is too heavy.
- Try to find a weight that feels moderately hard to lift around the eighth rep. Then try to get one or two more reps without compromising form (normally this means without rounding your back).
- Do three sets of eight to ten reps on each body part you are working. Rest for two minutes between sets.
- A good rule of thumb is to alternate upper body exercises and lower body exercises every other day. This way you give each muscle group a chance to recover before working it again.
- Lifting weights two to four times per week is plenty.

2. *Focus on whole foods*

As we age our metabolisms slow down. The more processed a food, the harder it will be for our body to use it for fuel. This means the body will tuck it away as a fat store. When I refer to whole foods, I am talking about foods that look the way they do in nature. For example a grain of rice on your plate looks like a grain of rice when it was in nature. But crackers made of rice flour no longer look like rice. Once again, always follow the conscious eating guidelines first. If rice crackers sound good and you are hungry, then eat them! But of course be mindful of how they make you feel. This strategy is more about adding in whole foods rather than taking anything out. If you are presented with choices and both sound equally appetizing, then opt for the whole food option. When cooking for yourself opt for whole foods when they sound good, stock them in your house, and have them ready to eat. Simple shifts, nothing dramatic or difficult to stick to!

There are certainly many supplements you can take that may help to some degree with changing hormone levels. There is nothing wrong with taking supplements or even seeing a doctor to investigate using hormone replacement therapy. Whenever you feel the desire arise to do something to slow down the natural aging process or the appearance of aging, tune into that and try to see where it is coming from. Is there fear of change, lack of self-acceptance, or a desire to go back to a previous time? Just pay attention and be sure to address the root of the desire for anti-aging whether or not you choose to take action against the symptoms of aging.

Conclusion

We live in a very exciting time in history. An increasing number of people are becoming conscious every day. And just in the nick of time. Our planet is suffering the consequences of humanity's collective unconsciousness. Unchecked consumption runs rampant as plastic fills our oceans and pollutants fill our air. Nature's purification systems are bogged down and can no longer keep up with the rate at which humans pollute the Earth. Interestingly enough, these same issues are mirrored in our own bodies. As overconsumption of food rises the body is unable to convert it into usable energy. The pancreas is overwhelmed and can no longer keep up with insulin production which gives rise to type II diabetes. It is not by chance that both individual bodies and our planet are showing the same signs of deterioration due to over consumption.

The similarities don't stop with overconsumption. In 2020 the United States of America as well as cities all over the world erupted with violent riots following the death of George Floyd and many other acts of racism and hate crimes. Racist acts are no doubt spurred by one group of people believing it is morally superior to another, even to the death. And at the same time we look at our social media feeds and wish we had her thighs or butt, judging them as better than ours. We look at someone passing by on the sidewalk and feel disgusted by the way their fat hangs off their arms. As much as we want to label someone else a "racist" and ourselves as "inclusive," until we can make the mental space to include our own cellulite and fat rolls our societies will continue to mirror our internal lack of unity.

Body Alchemy is lifesaving work. When we end the internal war, we do the work of ending all war. When compassion, respect, mindfulness, gentleness, boundaries, collaboration, self-worth and joy become the values that align our internal compasses, then rest assured the compass of greater society will fall into alignment as well. It is not by waging war on our bodies that we will become conquerors in possession of thin thighs. It is by deeply listening to the body and responding with compassion to its requests that ultimately leads to harmony and health.

Bodies are physical expressions of an invisible consciousness. This consciousness is our truest nature, not the body that houses it. We are indeed unique expressions of a central consciousness. Some might call this consciousness God. When we get still enough, and with enough practice, we can hear our truest nature, our God nature, speaking. And when we are brave enough to follow that voice, we align ourselves with the greatest power available. This is when finances, relationships, and yes, bodies, take their optimal form.

I now invite you to give up your wars one at a time and tap into the deep wisdom that is just below the tumultuous surface. Drop the fight and embrace who it is you were called here to be. Lose the nice girl disguise, stop following the advice of mental chatter, let emotions inform your path and boldly step into the human you were made to be. And then sit back and watch as your body takes the shape it was made to have.

www.ingramcontent.com/pod-product-compliance
Lightning Source LLC
Chambersburg PA
CBHW072300260726
48658CB00004BA/1330